INTRODUCTION
TO
ULTRASONOGRAPHY
AND
PATIENT CARE

▼

INTRODUCTION TO ULTRASONOGRAPHY AND PATIENT CARE

Marveen Craig, RDMS

W. B. SAUNDERS COMPANY

Harcourt Brace Jovanovich, Inc.

Philadelphia · London · Toronto · Montreal · Sydney · Tokyo

W. B. SAUNDERS COMPANY
Harcourt Brace Jovanovich, Inc.

The Curtis Center
Independence Square West
Philadelphia, Pennsylvania 19106

Library of Congress Cataloging-in-Publication Data
Craig, Marveen.
Introduction to ultrasonography and patient care / Marveen Craig.
   p. cm.
ISBN 0-7216-4229-2
1. Diagnosis, Ultrasonic.   I. Title.
  [DNLM: 1. Ultrasonography. WB 289 C886i]
RC78.7.U4C68 1993   616.07′543 – dc20
DNLM/DLC   91-46871

INTRODUCTION TO ULTRASONOGRAPHY   ISBN   0-7216-4229-2
AND PATIENT CARE

Printed in Mexico

Last digit is the print number: 9   8   7   6   5   4   3   2   1

To
ELIZABETH DIENES,
who nurtured the seed
from which this book has grown.

"Never regard study as a duty, but as the enviable opportunity to learn . . . "

Albert Einstein

Preface

There's never been a better time to be a sonographer! As we learn and grow, and find our place in the profession of diagnostic medical ultrasound, we have much to take pride in and much to look forward to.

New applications of medical sonography are constantly emerging and producing a growing demand for sonography services. As a result, new levels have appeared on the sonography career ladder that wouldn't have been thought of 20 years ago: clinical specialists, educators, entrepreneurial free-lance sonographers, applications specialists, and directors of research and development and product management.

The need for better educated, well-trained sonographers has never been greater, but it is no longer sufficient simply to study anatomy and physiology and to understand routine sonography principles and procedures. As a self-taught sonographer, I've experienced the frustration of digging for answers to the questions of the moment when textbooks and other common educational resources were not yet available.

While watching our field of diagnostic ultrasound come of age, it has become increasingly evident that ours is one diagnostic technique that cannot be learned and practiced by rote. It requires practitioners with intellectual curiosity and tenacity, discipline and interpersonal skills, and the recognition that the patient is the centerpiece of our endeavors.

With this in mind, I have tried to provide a set of hints that seemed to me to be useful—in hopes that they will add to the progress and enjoyment of the reader. This book was written not only for beginning students and teachers but also for veteran sonographers, and its objective is to assist in developing their heads, hands, and hearts, for these are the essence of a superior sonographer.

Marveen Craig

Acknowledgments

This book could not have come to fruition without the expert assistance of many talented individuals along the way. Although it is impossible to name them all, special recognition should go to

— **Lisa Biello**, without whom none of my books would have seen publication. Her encouragement, professional guidance, and unerring good taste make her my favorite editor.

— two unsung heroes: my son **Greg Lawrence**, who provides so much more than photography, illustrations, and computer guidance, and my husband **Walter**, who continues to surround me with love and support during all of my endeavors.

— my nursing school instructors, who unknowingly shaped my beliefs. I think they would be amazed.

— and the multitude of colleagues and students with whom I've been privileged to work. I want them to know that they are the heartbeat of this book.

TECHNICAL CONSULTANTS

Unit 4

John C. Pope, III, BS, RDMS
Cardiovascular Associates of Augusta
Augusta, Georgia

Unit 6

Sandra M. Karol, MA, RT, RDMS
Program Director, Sonography
Palm Beach Community College
Palm Beach Gardens, Florida

Contents

▼

U N I T   1

Foundations

Definitions and Origins of Diagnostic Medical Sonography

LEARNING OBJECTIVES

Students who successfully complete this unit will be able to:

- *Define* the following terms: sound and acoustics, ultrasound and ultrasonics, and diagnostic medical sonography.

- *Identify* some of the pioneers who shaped the new technology.

- *Describe* the evolutionary history of diagnostic medical sonography.

Diagnostic medical sonography is a relatively new profession in the ancient field of patient care. In many ways this medical prodigy is still evolving, inasmuch as major technologic breakthroughs and clinical applications continue to emerge at an astonishing rate.

Those who choose a career in sonography will become allied with the most modern use of sound in medical diagnosis. They will be required to master scientific principles and technical skills and to cultivate professionalism toward and empathy for their patients.

It is appropriate to undertake that quest by mastering basic terms and developing an understanding and appreciation of the origins and history of diagnostic medical sonography.

1

DEFINITIONS

The study of the science, engineering, and art of generating, propagating, and receiving sound waves is called *acoustics* (Academic American Encyclopedia, 1988). As a sonographer you will deal exclusively with *ultrasound,* the sound with frequencies beyond the upper limits of perception by the human ear (from approximately 2 to 20 kHz) (Dorland, 1988). Although ultrasonic radiation can be injurious to human tissues because of its thermal effects when absorbed by living matter, it can be used either therapeutically (in controlled doses) to selectively break down diseased tissues or diagnostically to visually display echoes received from irradiated tissues.

Diagnostic medical ultrasonography, or *sonography,* is an imaging technique used to visualize the deep tissue structures of the body by recording the returning reflections of ultrasonic waves directed into the body (Dorland, 1988). The terms often are used interchangeably.

Because the fledgling field of diagnostic ultrasound grew so quickly and contributions came from such varied sources, little time initially was expended on establishing terminology. This oversight resulted in a proliferation of terms and jargon — some borrowed (correctly and incorrectly) from other scientific disciplines and some invented out of sheer necessity. Universal agreement and acceptance of terminology have yet to be achieved, although progress is being made through the work of the Standards Committee of the American Institute of Ultrasound in Medicine. In this text the terms *ultrasonography* and *diagnostic ultrasonography* are used most often to describe the profession. The term *sonologist* is used to describe the physician who interprets the ultrasound study, whereas the term *sonographer* describes the individual who performs the ultrasound examination. Finally, the term *sonogram* is used interchangeably to indicate either the ultrasound examination itself or the hard-copy images produced during the examination.

HISTORICAL PERSPECTIVE

The tap roots of diagnostic ultrasonography can be traced to one of the oldest sciences — that of sound, or acoustics — which dates back to the ancient Greeks. However, the goal of this chapter is to acquaint the student with some of the contributing pioneers who shaped this new science rather than to provide a detailed history of ultrasound.

The Nature of Sound

The systematic study of sound began in 500 BC, with the Greek mathematician, Pythagoras, who observed the relationship between sound pitch and frequency. But much earlier cultures, such as those of the Egyptians, the Persians, and the Chinese, had developed musical instruments and become interested in the propagation of sound. Pythagoras is said to have invented the *sonometer,* an instrument used to study musical sounds (Academic American Encyclopedia, 1988).

One hundred years later, the Greek scholar Archytas of Tarentum defined the nature of sound, deducing that sound is produced by the motion of one object striking another – with swift motion producing a high pitch and slow motion producing a low pitch (Encyclopedia Americana, 1991). It was not until 350 BC that Aristotle developed the theory of sound propagation, that is, that sound is carried to the ears by the movement of air.

A familiar sound analogy, still used by contemporary physics teachers, can be attributed to the Roman philosopher Boethius, who was the first to compare sound waves to the waves produced by dropping a pebble into a calm body of water (Encyclopedia Americana, 1991; Encyclopaedia Brittanica, 1981).

From then until 1300 AD, little scientific investigation took place in Europe, although scientists in the Middle East and India were developing new ideas about sound by studying music and working out systems of music theory.

The study of sound remained relatively dormant during the Middle Ages but experienced a revival in the upsurge of scientific interest after the Renaissance period.

In 1500 the illustrious Leonardo da Vinci became intrigued with the physical properties of sound, and he is thought to have originated the idea that sound travels in waves. He also is credited with discovering that the angle of reflection is equal to the angle of incidence (Encyclopedia Americana, 1991).

Europeans did not begin extensive experiments on the nature of sound until 1638, when Galileo demonstrated that the frequency of sound waves determines pitch (Academic American Encyclopedia, 1988). In the late 1600s, Sir Isaac Newton announced the derivation of the theory of velocity, and the English chemist Robert Boyle popularized the theory of the elasticity of air (Encyclopedia Americana, 1991).

Over the next two and a half centuries, experiments would be performed and mathematic calculations developed that would lead to the current understanding of the fundamentals of acoustics. The end of the nineteenth century marked the beginning of the modern study of acoustics, with the publication of *Theory of Sound* (1877) by the British scientist, Lord Rayleigh. In his remarkable book, he gathered, clarified, and expanded the current knowledge of acoustics (Academic American Encyclopedia, 1988).

The Nature of Ultrasound

One of the first experiments dealing with ultrasound occurred in 1793, when Lazzaro Spallanzani, an Italian priest-scientist, studied the activities of bats. Observing that bats could function effectively in the dark even if blinded — but not if deafened — Spallanzani theorized that the bats were listening to something he could not hear. Exactly what it was eluded him (Encyclopedia Americana, 1991; Goldberg, 1988; Knight, 1980; Scott, 1973).

During the scientifically rich nineteenth century, theories, investigations, and discoveries about sound abounded. Among them were the theory of wave diffraction proposed by the French physicist Augustin Fresnel, the invention of the ultrasonic whistle by Sir Francis Galton, and the description of the ferromagnetic effect by James Joule (Encyclopedia Americana, 1991).

The effect of motion on the pitch of sounds was first postulated by the Austrian scientist Christian Johann Doppler and named the *Doppler effect* in his honor. Even Wilhelm Röntgen was involved in studying sound before x-rays captured his attention (Encyclopaedia Brittanica, 1983; Encyclopedia Americana, 1991; Encyclopedia of the Biological Sciences, 1970; Goldberg, 1988).

The field of ultrasound was made accessible, however, in 1880, with the discovery by the Curie brothers (Jacques and Pierre) of the phenomenon of piezoelectricity. These researchers established the presence of the piezoelectric effect when they observed that certain crystals would expand and contract slightly when placed in an alternating electrical field. Reverse piezoelectricity permitted the same crystal to create an electrical potential, or voltage, making the crystals useful as both receivers and sources of sound waves, from audible to ultrasonic frequencies (Academic American Encyclopedia, 1988; Encyclopaedia Brittanica, 1983; Encyclopedia Americana, 1991; Encyclopedia of the Biological Sciences, 1970; Goldberg, 1988). Their accomplishments ultimately led to development of the modern ultrasound transducer.

In 1845 Doppler formulated his principle — that when a source of wave motion itself moves, the apparent frequency of the emitted waves changes (Academic American Encyclopedia, 1988; Encyclopedia Americana, 1991; Goldberg, 1988; Knight, 1980).

Not until the twentieth century did scientists learn how to produce ultrasound and how to put it to work. Until then ultrasonic waves were little more than a scientific curiosity.

In the early 1900s, piezoelectric transducers were used in an early form of sonar to detect the presence of submarines.

During World War I, French scientist Paul Langevin, who was studying controlled sound frequency and intensity, discovered a way to use the property of echoing sound waves to detect underwater objects. His discoveries came too late for military use, but he unknowingly laid the groundwork for the development of sonar in the next great war (Academic American Encyclopedia, 1988; Encyclopaedia Brittanica, 1981; Encyclopedia Americana, 1991; Encyclopedia of Biological Sciences, 1970; Goldberg, 1988; World Book Encyclopedia, 1991). Langevin also discovered the effect of ultrasound on marine life when he observed that small fish swimming through ultrasound beams were killed instantly. He realized the potential power of the energy with which he was dealing when one of his assistants, holding his hand in the path of the sound wave for only a brief instant, experienced agonizing pain—"as if the very bones were being heated!" (Goldberg, 1988).

The answer to Spallanzani's eighteenth century questions had to wait until 1938, when G. W. Pierce invented a sonic detector. This instrument was able to pick up the very high frequency vibrations of bats and to convert them into audible sounds (Scott, 1973).

Science and industry are jointly responsible for the great strides made in the understanding and refinement of ultrasonic energy. Industrialists such as Floyd Firestone, with his ultrasonic machine called the *Reflectoscope,* harnessed its awesome power and found many uses for it such as metallic flaw detection and cleansing (Goldberg, 1988; Holmes, 1980).

MEDICAL APPLICATIONS

The destructive nature of ultrasound on biologic organisms and living tissues was first discussed by Robert Williams Wood and Alfred Lee Loomis in 1927 (Encyclopaedia of Biological Sciences, 1970). The effect of high doses of ultrasonic energy on the body is as injurious as x-rays and atomic radiation. In lower doses, however, it can be a therapeutic agent. The effects produced by high-energy ultrasonic waves normally are irreversible and arise from cavitation, intense mechanical stresses, or intense localized heating. Focused ultrasound waves are used to remove unwanted tissue. The minimum ultrasound dose is not easily defined at present, nor is it possible to correlate a definite type of tissue damage with a universally standardized dosage (Encyclopaedia Brittanica, 1983; Encyclopedia of the Biological Sciences, 1970).

In contrast, low-intensity ultrasonic waves can be used to visualize the interior of the body. An ultrasonic examination is noninvasive, and since the late 1960s, scientists have been painlessly probing the soft tissues of the human body — seeing with sound.

In 1942, in Austria, Karl Dussik was one of the first physicians to utilize ultrasound for diagnostic purposes. He claimed that tumors of the brain could be detected by the ultrasonic mapping of the attenuation of sound in brain tissues, and he called these maps (produced by means of amplitude modulation or A-mode techniques) *hyperphonograms* (Goldberg, 1988; Holmes, 1980).

The development of metal flaw detectors and naval sonar also made possible the work of three independent American investigators: George Ludwig, John Wild, and Douglass Howry.

From 1947 to 1949, Ludwig, a Pennsylvania surgeon, working first at the Naval Medical Research Institute and then with colleagues at the Massachusetts Institute of Technology, successfully used ultrasound to detect gallstones (Goldberg, 1988; Holmes, 1980) (Fig. 1–1).

Wild, an English surgeon who emigrated to Minnesota, first thought of using ultrasound to detect tissue thickness. In his work at the University of Minnesota, he came to realize that cancerous tissues differed greatly from normal tissues. Along with John Reid, he constructed an early prototype breast scanner that employed the use of an externally placed water path (Fig. 1–2). Wild also was a pioneer in the development of early internal scanners, devising a rectal transducer to obtain images of the large bowel (Goldberg, 1988; Holmes, 1980).

At the same time, in Denver, Colorado, Howry, working independently of the other groups and using war surplus electronic components, devised a "water-path" scanner. He also used a laundry tub and later a cattle tank for his first prototypes, in which the subject or body part to be imaged was submersed in water (Fig. 1–3). The resulting one-dimensional images, however, were disappointingly incomplete. Joining forces with Joseph Holmes, University of Colorado physician and professor, he developed a compound scanner (Goldberg, 1988; Holmes, 1980). Howry and Holmes discovered that by

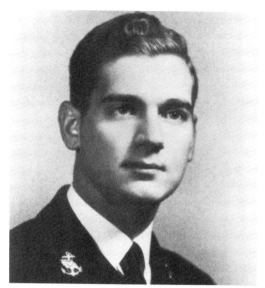

A

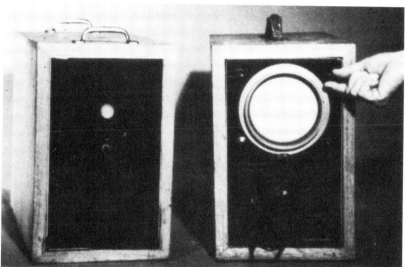

B

Figure 1–1. *A,* **George D. Ludwig.** Ludwig conducted A-mode experiments for the U.S. Navy to detect the presence of gallstones and other foreign bodies embedded in animal tissues. One of his primary concerns was establishing the physical and physiological standards of the velocity of ultrasonic transmission through gallstones vs. tissue. *B,* Scanning apparatus used by Dr. Ludwig to investigate sound transmission and the acoustic properties of tissue. *(Reprinted courtesy Eastman Kodak Company.)*

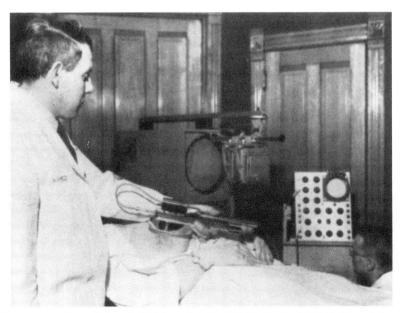

Figure 1–2. Drs. John A. Wild and John M. Reid. Dr. Wild *(left)* applying a B-mode scanner to a patient's breast, while Dr. Reid operates the system controls *(lower right). (Reprinted courtesy Eastman Kodak Company.)*

moving the transducer in two different motion patterns simultaneously, a more complete anatomic picture could be formed. The cattle tank eventually was replaced by a B-29 gun turret, and the subject not only was immersed but also was weighted down to avoid floating or motion artifacts as the mechanically circling transducer cut a path through the water (Fig. 1–4).

The impracticality of using this procedure with sick patients spurred these scientists to simplify the procedure and to successfully develop a "pan" scanner that permitted the patient to sit next to, but outside, a small pan of water through which the transducer moved.

The experience Howry and Holmes gained eventually led to the development of a compound contact scanner, which permitted direct scanning of the body with the use of a light film of oil or lubricating gel to replace the cumbersome water-path (Fig. 1–5).

Holmes worked closely with William Wright, an electronic engineer, after Howry left Denver to work at the Massachusetts Institute of Technology. The fruits of their labors were realized in 1962, with the introduction of the first commercially available Physionics Engineering Porta-arm compound contact scanner, a portable, ultrasonic system (Goldberg, 1988; Holmes, 1980) (Fig. 1–6).

In the mid-1950s, at the University of Glasgow, Ian Donald began his studies of diagnostic ultrasonography. His interest developed as a result of his World War II experiences with the Royal Air Force, during which he witnessed the ultrasonic testing of aircraft to detect

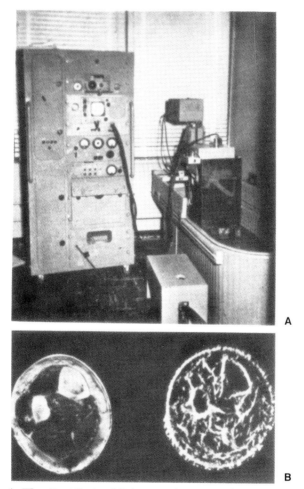

A

B

Figure 1–3. *A,* **The "cattle-tank" immersion scanning system.** Note the transducer assembly mounted on the wooden track running along the outside edge of the tank. The actual transducer was submerged within the water-filled tank. *B,* Horizontal ultrasonic scan of a human leg produced by the cattle-tank scanner. *(Reprinted courtesy Eastman Kodak Company.)*

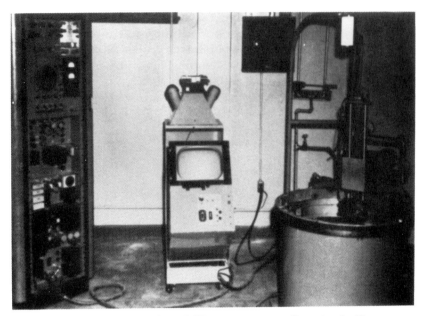

Figure 1–4. Howry and Holmes' "B-29 gun turret" water-bath scanner (c. 1953–1954). Note the transducer assembly mounted on a ring encircling the tank. This arrangement provided a complete 360 degree scan-path around the immersed patient. The transducer could be raised and lowered to a desired level within the tank. A second motor moved the transducer in a four-inch back-and-forth sectoring motion. The tall console on the left contained the electronic system, the display console is seen in the center, and the gun turret and transducer carriage assembly are seen on the right. *(Reprinted courtesy Eastman Kodak Company.)*

metal stress and fatigue. Donald vowed to pursue his notion that ultrasound might be used in a similar fashion on patients (Goldberg, 1988; Holmes, 1980).

By means of a comparative examination of a tumor and a beefsteak, Donald proved that tumors possessed echo patterns different from those of normal tissue. This work was conducted in an atomic boiler plant outside Glasgow with use of a borrowed flaw detector. Later, again using borrowed equipment and A-mode technique, he began detecting ovarian cysts, ascites, and polyhydramnios in patients (Goldberg, 1988; Holmes, 1980). Donald ultimately perfected the ultrasonic A-mode measurement of the biparietal diameter of the fetal head, making it possible to estimate fetal age, weight, and growth rate.

In 1957 Donald collaborated with an industrial engineer, Tom Brown, to develop a contact compound scanner. They mounted it on a bedside table and suspended it over the patient. Manipulating the transducer by hand underneath the table, Donald, using brightness modulation (B-mode) technique, produced the first crude fetal scans. By 1960 Donald and Brown had developed a mechanical sector scanner and later a hand-held scanner called the *Diasonograph,* suit-

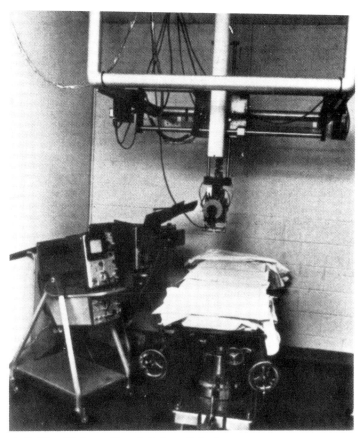

Figure 1–5. The University of Colorado's first compound contact scanner. (Constructed by consulting engineers William Wright and Ed Meyer for Dr. Joseph Holmes.) The system required one individual to manually guide the ceiling-mounted transducer carriage across the patient's body, as the transducer mechanically sectored 30 degrees to either side of the perpendicular. A second individual operated the controls and the camera seen on the left. It was this system that was used during the 1960s to develop many of the scanning protocols still practiced today. *(Reprinted courtesy Eastman Kodak Company.)*

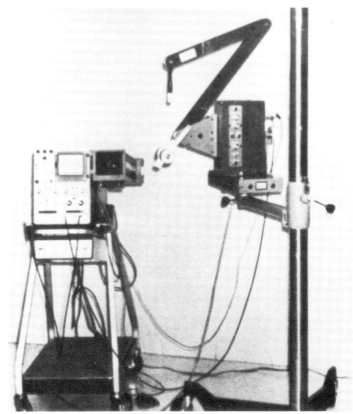

Figure 1–6. Porta-arm Scanner. Engineers Wright and Meyer developed this portable compound contact scanner after forming their own company: Physionics Engineering. Freed from the ceiling mount and positioned upon a wheeled tripod, the transducer mechanism, a 3-jointed scanning arm, and a mechanical and electronic "box" could be moved along a calibrated metal track. Horizontal or longitudinal positioning of the "arm" permitted scans in two planes. A single operator could now operate scanner, controls, and camera. *(Reprinted courtesy Eastman Kodak Company.)*

able for commercial distribution (Goldberg, 1988; Holmes, 1980) (Fig. 1–7).

Despite Donald's involvement in the research and development of ultrasound equipment, his primary interest was in applying diagnostic ultrasonography to his specialty of obstetrics and gynecology (Fig. 1–8). He is credited with contributing to the diagnosis of multiple pregnancies, hydramnios, hydatidiform mole, and the introduction of the fluid-filled bladder technique used in early pregnancy and gynecologic studies. His crowning achievement occurred in 1954 when he was the first to demonstrate a fetal gestational sac, which earned him the title "father of obstetrical ultrasound" (Goldberg, 1988).

The year 1954 witnessed another exciting discovery. In Sweden, physicist Carl Hellmuth Hertz and Dr. Inge Edler, using a flaw detector borrowed from the Malmö shipyards, demonstrated a *motion display* of the heart and intracardiac structures. Employing the use of both A- and B-mode techniques, they added a continuously moving display of the returning cardiac echoes (Fig. 1–9). At first they were stymied by an inability to identify the various motion patterns, until Edler established the characteristic motion patterns for the anterior leaflet of the mitral valve. Edler's observations were

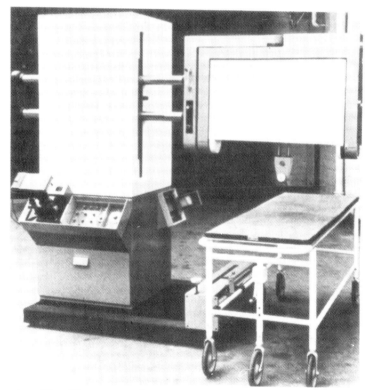

Figure 1–7. The Diasonograph. Developed from prototypes designed by Donald and Brown, the Diasonograph was introduced commercially by Nuclear Enterprises, Ltd., Edinburgh, in 1964. *(Reprinted courtesy Eastman Kodak Company.)*

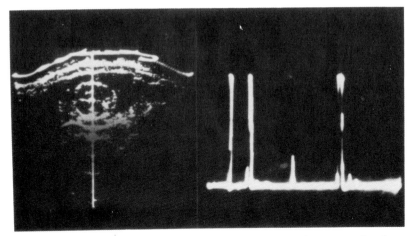

Figure 1–8. Fetal head and biparietal measurement. A cross-sectional scan of the fetal head outlined in B-mode presentation appears on the *left*. An A-mode presentation of the midline echo appears on the *right*. This scan (c. 1964) is thought to have been produced with the Diasonograph. *(Reprinted courtesy Eastman Kodak Company.)*

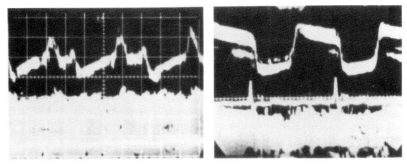

Figure 1–9. Early M-mode scans of the mitral valve. Hertz and Edler developed an ultrasonic technique to display graphic cardiac motion. Reflected echo information appeared as a bright dot moving along the screen as the structure being imaged moved or shifted position. A special camera and continuous moving film displayed the wave form motion of the echo dot reflected from the intracardiac structures. Normal mitral valve patterns are seen on the *left*. An abnormal, flat-topped stenotic mitral valve pattern is seen on the *right*. *(Reprinted courtesy Eastman Kodak Company.)*

later validated by Dr. Sven Effert, who placed a transducer directly on the heart, verifying all of Edler's previous identification and motion patterns. With this achievement the diagnostic potential of echocardiography became apparent (Goldberg, 1988). Construction of echocardiography equipment would not take place, however, until cardiologist Claude Joyner and engineer John Reid at the University of Pennsylvania collaborated with Howry and Holmes at the University of Colorado (Goldberg, 1988; Holmes, 1980).

Early ophthalmologic ultrasound applications were pioneered by Arvo Oksala in Finland and Gilbert Baum in the United States during the 1950s. Oksala was the first to adapt A-mode technique for use in the eye and to correctly interpret the resulting echocardiographic data (Goldberg, 1988; Knight, 1980).

Baum initially worked with the A-mode presentation, but dissatisfied with its lack of precision, he turned his efforts to applying B-mode techniques to ophthalmology. Baum and his colleagues were the first to employ ultrasonic frequencies of 10 to 15 MHz, which produced significantly higher resolution. Baum also was successful in producing a three-dimensional image of the eyes with what he called "third-generation" B-mode ultrasound equipment. The system employed succeeding scans at each millimeter of eye depth (Goldberg, 1988).

A dramatic application of ultrasonography in ophthalmic medicine took place in the late 1960s, when Dr. Nathaniel Bronson, working in New York City, combined two new medical developments. The first was a tiny forceps that could grasp very small objects easily and accurately. The other discovery was spurred by a suggestion by the aforementioned Finnish scientist, Arvo Oksala, to use a sonar beam to "see" inside the eye (Knight, 1980).

Using war surplus electronic components, Bronson assembled a sonar device that could explore the eye from the outside. Then he devised a hand-held, combination sonar transducer-probe, small enough to operate inside the minuscule incisions used in eye surgery. Hooking the probe up to a small oscilloscope screen to display the echoes, Bronson tested the probe on every bit of foreign matter that could conceivably lodge in the human eye (Goldberg, 1988; Knight, 1980). In September of 1964 at Walter Reed Hospital, outside Washington, D.C., Bronson's device was used successfully on a human being for the first time to remove a 1/4-inch brass sliver from the eye of an 11-year-old boy (Knight, 1980; Sochurek, 1988).

The 1950s and 1960s were to become the golden age of diagnostic ultrasonography. Australian engineer George Kossoff, with the help of T. Garrett, constructed a compound water-path scanner for obstetric use. He also pioneered in the development of gray-scale imaging, which dramatically increased the information content of images and revolutionized diagnostic ultrasonographic equipment design and acceptance (Goldberg, 1988).

Japanese work in diagnostic ultrasonography, which began in 1950, roughly paralleled the developments taking place in Europe and the United States. Considerably more emphasis was placed on Doppler examination of the heart by the Japanese than by scientists in any other country. Also, at the same time that Kossoff and Garrett were perfecting their water-path scanner, physicist Rokuru Uchida and Dr. S. Oka were building a special apparatus for a new ultrasound application: the shattering of renal stones (Goldberg, 1988; Holmes, 1980).

It was not until the late 1950s that serious Doppler ultrasound research was undertaken. Robert Rushmer and Dean Franklin at the University of Washington in Seattle were joined in 1958 by Donald Baker, who designed several sophisticated, implantable flowmeters. The Seattle group is credited with the development of a small hand-held portable, continuous-wave Doppler device for transcutaneous use. In 1964, Eugene Strandness, a vascular surgery resident, joined the group to conduct clinical trials. His involvement with the project caused him to devote his career to the study and development of noninvasive measuring of the peripheral vascular systems. A giant step forward came with his 1967 publication on assigning particular waveforms to specific disease conditions (Strandness et al., 1967).

Work on pulsed Doppler applications began in 1966 and culminated in the development of the first pulsed Doppler system by Baker and co-worker, Dennis Watkins (with guidance from John Reid) (Goldberg, 1988).

The role of Doppler ultrasonography continues to unfold, with color Doppler displays simplifying the understanding of blood flow physiology and presenting yet another intricate piece to the puzzle of medical diagnosis.

The biophysical and therapeutic applications of ultrasound have a longer history than do the applications of ultrasound for diagnosis. Among the major contributors to the understanding of its applications in biology and medicine were William Fry, a physicist at the University of Illinois, and his brother, Francis Fry, who founded the Bioacoustics Research Laboratory. William Fry, aided by a Navy research grant, explored the possibilities that high-intensity ultrasound eventually could provide a noninvasive, lower-risk surgical technique, as compared with standard invasive surgery. He was to find that it also would offer unique advantages in the investigation of how the brain functioned. Fry designed a sophisticated system employing a multiple transducer system of focused, high-intensity sound beams that could produce a pinpoint lesion without damage to surrounding tissue (Goldberg, 1988; Holmes, 1980). Francis Fry later became interested in developing a computer-based, low-intensity ultrasound instrument for soft tissue visualization. With his co-worker, Elizabeth Kelly, he embarked on the study of use of ultrasound for detecting breast cancer. Elizabeth Kelly Fry is recognized today as one of the leading authorities on ultrasonic breast scanning.

SUMMARY

The fortieth anniversary of diagnostic medical sonography was observed in 1988. The modality has continued to advance enormously for the last 20 years—from the introduction of real-time imaging (which brought dynamic movement to the previously static B-mode images) in 1973 to the continuing technologic breakthroughs that have resulted in high-resolution transducers, two-dimensional or 2-D echocardiography (demonstration of the heart as a moving structure by means of the real-time B-mode technique), and endocorporeal and invasive transducer techniques. Diagnostic ultrasound has indeed far exceeded many of its pioneers' expectations.

The infant is coming of age. What will tomorrow bring? The results remain to be seen, but judging by past history and performance, the prospects are extraordinarily promising. They promise to be not only evolutionary but also revolutionary.

REFERENCES

1. Academic American Encyclopedia, 1st ed., s.v. "sound and acoustics." Danbury, Conn.: Grolier, Inc., 1988.
2. Dorland's Illustrated Medical Dictionary, 27th ed., Philadelphia: W. B. Saunders, 1988.
3. Encyclopedia Americana, International ed., s.v. "sound." Danbury, Conn.: Grolier Inc., 1991.
4. Encyclopaedia Brittanica, 15th ed., s.v. "sound." Chicago: Encyclopaedia Brittanica, Inc., 1983.
5. Encyclopedia of the Biological Sciences, 2nd ed., s.v. "ultrasonics." New York: Van Norstrand Reinhold Co., 1981.
6. Goldberg, B. B.: Medical Diagnostic Ultrasound: A Retrospective on its 40th Anniversary. Bethesda, Md.: American Institute of Ultrasound in Medicine, 1988.

7. Holmes, J. H.: Diagnostic ultrasound during the early years of A.I.U.M. Journal of Clinical Ultrasound 1980; 8(4):299-308.

8. Knight, D. C.: Silent Sound. The World of Ultrasonics. New York: William Morrow & Co., 1980.

9. Scott, J. M.: What Is Sound? New York: Parents' Press, 1973.

10. Sochurek, H.: Medicine's New Vision. Easton, Penn.: Mack Publishing Co., 1988.

11. Strandness, D. E., Schultz, R. D., Sumner, D. S., and Rushmer, R. F.: Ultrasonic flow detection—A useful technic in the evaluation of peripheral vascular disease. American Journal of Surgery 1967; 113:311.

U N I T 2

Orientation

Anatomy of a Sonographer

LEARNING OBJECTIVES

Students who successfully complete this unit will be able to:

- Define the role of the sonographer.
- List specific aptitudes, abilities, and skills desirable in sonographer candidates.
- Compare and contrast the pros and cons of a sonography career.
- Name two resource organizations devoted specifically to sonographers.

The past two decades have produced a marked growth in the field of allied health careers. This growth has occurred partly because the proliferation of medical technologic advances that took place during that time created a critical need for professionals adept at using new and complex instruments.

The "high-tech" era also has added new dimensions to the practice of medicine, as advanced research techniques promote the discovery of new causes and cures for diseases. It has encouraged the concept of physician specialization, and in so doing has provided room for expanding the role of allied health professionals to one of physician assistant.

At first glance the day-to-day practice of sonography appears deceptively simple. On closer inspection and exposure to the process, it becomes apparent that sonographers face a workday filled with complex challenges. Such exposure also makes it apparent that the transducer-wielding sonographer has a profound effect on the quality of an examination and that in-depth education and training are required to achieve the greatest possible diagnostic benefits.

With every advance in technology, sonographers are expected to develop skills that might not have been part of their training programs even five years ago. Such skills as increased expertise in patient care, pathophysiology, and computer literacy, added to rapid and ongoing instrumentation changes, can be both exciting and frustrating.

THE ROLE OF SONOGRAPHER

Role is a specific behavior that an individual demonstrates to others; *function,* on the other hand, involves the tasks or duties one is obligated to perform in carrying out a role.

The term *sonographer* literally means one who graphs or draws with sound. A sonographer performs ultrasound studies and gathers diagnostic data under the direct or indirect supervision of a physician. The sonographer's role, however, is more than tasks delegated by physicians. Sonography is a unique profession with its own theoretic basis. Not only do sonographers provide care, using the most up-to-date equipment available, but they also touch their patients, not only with their hands but with their hearts. To be a good sonographer today, it is necessary not only to possess strong scientific knowledge and skills but to work diligently to keep abreast of the field and also to cultivate tender care and concern for one's patients.

QUALITIES OF A SONOGRAPHER

What specific aptitudes, abilities, and skills are indicative of a good sonographer? To answer that question, it is important to realize that aptitudes are not skills or abilities but rather undeveloped and untrained talents. The possession of an aptitude produces a natural tendency to do well. The following categories list some of the most desirable sonographer qualities.

Intellectual curiosity. Sonographers should be intrigued by science and challenged by the thought of putting it to work to help people. A paramedical background or clinical expertise is a requirement for entering the field. Eventually, many sonographers become interested in teaching or research, or both.

Eagerness and perseverance. Candidates for sonography training must be willing to attend an academic program beyond high school level and be ready to spend untold hours studying. Sonographers are required to take mathematics and scientific courses and to be able to integrate that knowledge in their clinical activities to produce better scans.

Quick-thinking and analytic capabilities. Sonographers must be capable of making accurate, independent judgments, because patients' lives may depend on them. The ability to plan and organize time and resources also are important traits, inasmuch as sonographers are expected to adapt the pace of an examination to fit prevailing needs.

Technical orientation. One of the most critical needs is the ability to conceptualize images in three-dimensional form and to possess good psychomotor skills. Sonographer candidates should be interested in working with their hands and with equipment—and constantly willing to learn new technical skills. In addition to adeptness in using many sophisticated machines and devices, sonographers must be adaptable and creative in those instances when equipment malfunctions.

Physical health. Good health is important because physical stamina is required for the hard work involved: long periods on one's feet, moving about, lifting and positioning patients, and performing other physically demanding tasks. Sonographers should be able to handle stress and be skilled in helping others cope with it.

Self-direction. Because sonography is never dull or routine, sonographers must be creative—able to "roll with the punches" and to make independent decisions. They should be capable of remaining unfrustrated by disruption of routine and be able to function autonomously.

Emotional stability. Sonographer candidates should be stimulated by the prospect of daily involvement in life and death situations. Not all examinations have happy endings, and often sonographers find themselves working with patients under great stress. It takes an emotionally stable person to be nurturing and compassionate in such situations.

Communication skills. Sonographers must be effective communicators as well as good listeners because they are frequently required to teach patients and family members, medical students, interns, and other sonographers. The ability to interact effectively with patients and medical personnel and to work as part of a team is critically important. Verbal communication skills and the competence to develop written reports also are necessary. A sonographer must feel comfortable in delegating tasks to co-workers and interacting with physicians and other health care personnel. As they move up through the ranks of the profession and are given more responsibilities, sonographers also need persuasive negotiating, leadership, and management skills.

Dedication. Sonographers should find satisfaction in working with all types of patients, including children, expectant mothers, and elderly persons. They should be sensitive and giving, as well as tenacious and flexible, as they seek the best results for their patients. Above all, they must be dedicated to their profession.

CAREER ADVANTAGES

Why become a sonographer? The greatest reward in sonography comes with the satisfaction of knowing that you were able to help a patient—that your skills and abilities made a difference. Another strong attraction of the field is respect. A good sonographer is treated as a competent resource person and is held in high esteem.

Being a member of a unique profession is a definite plus, as is the freedom to express creativity, authority, and judgment. It is highly satisfying to work one-on-one with patients, to tailor a study to the individual patient, and to deliver personalized patient care.

The diversity of career options offered in sonography also exerts a magnetic effect. The variety of specialties to choose from, the fact that day-to-day work is so vastly different, and the opportunity to obtain employment anywhere in the world are strong attractions. Attractive salaries and the flexibility of designing work hours to fit personal requirements (e.g., part-time vs. full-time work and shared jobs) are other benefits.

The field of sonography offers rich human experiences and is never dull. Although it is often stressful and demanding, the opportunities to solve problems and to meet professional challenges are personally rewarding.

The thing that makes medicine appealing is its reverence for life—its power and sacredness. The integration of science into this mystery is exciting. Searching for pieces of a puzzle that do not fit perfectly and then working to restore the balance bring a great sense of accomplishment. Although individual situations may require only a one-time use of their medical skill, sonographers require an understanding of many facets of disease to make good decisions. Thus the field allows them to satisfy their intellectual curiosity while serving humanity.

In addition to a consideration of a profession's advantages, it is equally important to evaluate its disadvantages. Accepting the challenge of professionalism often means accepting the fact that there may be no cure for a particular disease and that some patients certainly will die. The only consolation in this case is the knowledge that a sonographer's concern and skill have improved the patient's quality of life and ultimately will influence the care of future patients.

Career sonography cannot be compared with traditional 9-to-5 jobs. Being a sonographer often means frustration, fatigue, and depression; however, for each frustration there is a small triumph. The profession does not appeal to everyone. Only the individual can decide whether he or she is equal to the challenge.

INFORMATION SOURCES

The evolution of sonography as a career has been almost as colorful as the field of diagnostic medical sonography itself. Early operators of ultrasonic equipment in the United States were medical students, interns, residents, and "research assistants" plucked from such unlikely workers as receptionists, secretaries, orderlies, teachers, and housewives, as well as from the fields of nursing and radiology.

Interest in ultrasound grew quickly, and to meet the demands for training, pioneering laboratories and commercial equipment manufacturers opened their doors to any interested observers. The transfer of technical knowledge occurred in a show-and-tell fashion as the number of "trained" technicians slowly increased. The allied health profession of sonography could not have developed without the aid of those early workers and the important ultrasound organizations described here.

American Institute of Ultrasound in Medicine

In August 1951, an organization to promote the use of ultrasound in physical medicine was formed. One year later, the group, calling itself the American Institute of Ultrasound in Medicine (AIUM), conducted its first annual meeting in conjunction with the American Congress of Physical Medicine. Initially, membership was open only to physiatrists, but by 1964 the AIUM welcomed all physicians and bioengineers interested in the medical applications of ultrasound, particularly those in the field of diagnosis.

Over the years the number of physiatrists declined, leaving the diagnostically oriented members in the majority. The organization has continued to flourish, and today the AIUM remains the primary multidisciplinary, nonprofit society dedicated to advancing the art and science of ultrasound in medicine and research. Its current membership of 8000 is composed of physicians, scientists, engineers, sonographers, technicians, manufacturers and manufacturers' representatives, and medical students working toward the professional, educational, research, and scientific needs of medical specialists practicing ultrasound in medicine.

Society of Diagnostic Medical Sonographers

In 1965 the AIUM invited interested ultrasound technicians to attend its scientific sessions until such time as the technicians could found their own technical society.

That event took place in 1970, with the formation of the American Society of Ultrasound Technical Specialists (ASUTS), with a total membership of six. The goal of the society was to promote, advance, and educate its members, as well as the medical community, in the science of diagnostic medical ultrasound and, as a consequence, to contribute to the enhancement of patient care. Within several years, membership had grown to several hundred technicians, and the ASUTS turned its efforts toward gaining recognition of ultrasound technology as a new health career.

On October 4, 1974, the American Medical Association (AMA) responded to a request by the ASUTS for the creation of a new and separate health occupation — and a new title: the Diagnostic Medical Sonographer. Under the guidance of the AMA, the ASUTS and other collaborating organizations developed a Document of Essentials, which set forth the minimum educational requirements for sonography training and which would serve as a guide to curriculum development in formal ultrasound educational programs.

For consistency with the new terminology, the name of the ASUTS was formally changed in 1978 to the Society of Diagnostic Medical Sonographers (SDMS). With a current membership of more than 6000, the SDMS continues to set high educational standards, to monitor the socioeconomic concerns of its membership, and to promote excellence in the field. Through the efforts of its Professional Status Committee, a code of conduct was adopted.

American Registry of Diagnostic Medical Sonographers

Recognizing that the new profession needed some way to evaluate and certify the proficiency of sonographers, the ASUTS formed an examination committee to explore the possibility of measuring the levels of competency of persons who perform various diagnostic ultrasound studies. Its goal was achieved in 1975, with the formation of the American Registry of Diagnostic Medical Sonographers (ARDMS). Each year this organization conducts certifying examinations for qualified sonographers, in each of the specialty areas of diagnostic ultrasound. Appropriate credentials (i.e., Registered Diagnostic Medical Sonographer) are awarded to those who successfully complete the examinations.

Although registration is a voluntary activity in all but a few states, registered sonographers, to maintain their registry status, must provide proof of 30 hours of continuing education each triennium.

Joint Review Committee–Diagnostic Medical Sonography

Upon completion of the Document of Essentials, the SDMS, again working with the AMA and other interested collaborating organizations, established the Joint Review Committee for Diagnostic Medical Sonography. The purpose of this group is to attend to the inspection, evaluation, and ultimate accreditation (under the auspices of the Committee on Allied Health Education and Accreditation [CAHEA]) of formal training programs in ultrasound technology.

SUMMARY

The term *sonographer,* like the discipline, is deceptively simple; no matter how sophisticated instrumentation becomes, without the expertise of the sonographer, the blips and echoes on the oscilloscope or TV monitor are merely electrical impulses being converted to light. Just as a sculptor can envision a form within raw material, so too do sonographers see valuable and critical information in the dancing electronic displays before them. Through their talents and intelligence they know when and how to produce the images that will enable physicians to convert those same dots and dashes of light into healing answers.

It is impossible to categorize sonographers within other allied health care areas. They are unique—straddling many career fields as they care for their patients, assess both clinical and ultrasound problems, and work diligently to create high-quality studies suitable for accurate diagnostic interpretation. "Versatile," "intellectually stimulated," "resilient," and "idealistic" are only a few of the adjectives that personify the new health professional called *the sonographer.*

▼

U N I T   3

The Sonographer As Student

Learning Dynamics, Testing, Educational Curricula, and Programs of Study

LEARNING OBJECTIVES

Students who successfully complete this unit will be able to:

- Identify the three methods of learning, each of which uses a different sense.
- Describe how to set up an appropriate study area at home.
- Discuss the different methods of taking notes while reading or listening to tapes or lectures.
- Name the steps in the *PQRST* method of note taking.
- Differentiate between objective and subjective tests.
- Explain the relationship between clinical education and the didactic components of the sonography curriculum.
- Discuss competencies commonly evaluated in clinical education.
- Describe the basic courses essential to the education of a diagnostic medical sonographer.
- Discuss the various types of educational and training options available to sonographers.

As one of imaging's most accessible instruments, diagnostic ultrasound has also rapidly become a broad-based instrument. Its appeal to a wide spectrum of specialty physicians and their patients has resulted in constantly increasing demands for competent sonologists and sonographers. Unfortunately, the current lack of nationally accepted and defined clinical and educational standards has permitted extreme variables in sonologist and sonographer education and training. Until training standards for both sonologists and sonographers are adopted in our country, sonographers must be apprised of this situation and be made aware that pressures and unrealistic expectations may await them as they enter the workplace. Consequently, they must learn not only how to operate ultrasonic equipment but how to distinguish normal from abnormal sonographic anatomy, to correlate pertinent clinical data, and to fully recognize their own technical and educational limitations as well as their strengths.

Regardless of your background in allied health education or the length of time you have been out of school, you will be learning many things besides sonographic technique. Some of you will learn about hospital rules and regulations for the first time and about the many ways of getting along with patients, staff members, and fellow students. Even if you are a veteran allied health professional, you may find yourself spending time struggling to understand new and unfamiliar medical terminology as you expand your knowledge of patient care and the need to correlate clinical information from patients' charts.

The goal of this chapter is to help you get the most out of your sonographer-student experience by first explaining the complex process of learning, by offering suggestions on the art of studying to learn, and by providing information on current educational options in the United States.

LEARNING DYNAMICS

Critical Thinking and Action

For many years the American educational model has been to "drill" students to memorize information rather than to understand it. Who can forget reciting the multiplication tables by rote, only to stumble through the concepts of long division?

Today, modern educators are calling for educational reform that will teach students how to think rather than to memorize and then forget. Educational methods now focus less on simply imparting facts and theories and more on developing students' capacities for judgment, fact gathering, analysis, and synthesis to prepare them to meet the educational and employment challenges of the 1990s and the next century.

Educating sonographers should be no different. Old habits die hard, however, and some students begin their sonography education expecting to be handed a master list of facts to memorize. Such students are doomed to frustration until they realize that working in the field of diagnostic medicine is a problem-solving activity, comparable to working on a complex jigsaw puzzle. Simply taking an inventory of all the puzzle pieces will not provide the answers. The key to a solution lies in observing how the shapes of individual pieces might interconnect with other pieces in various areas of the puzzle. Only through trial and error and by blending experience (memory) and logic (reasoning) can difficult puzzles be solved correctly.

Memory

Each of us has three completely different types of memory: *immediate memory, short-term memory,* and *long-term memory* (Cermak, 1975). Immediate memory is for instantaneous use, whereas short-term memory usually is reserved for the temporary storage of facts — only long enough to use them — because they quickly fade. In contrast, long-term memory allows the permanent storage of information that is to be used (often repeatedly) over lengthy periods of time.

Immediate memory is the least understood and most often overlooked of the three systems; it is employed to remember things only long enough to respond to them. Reading this page is an example of immediate memory. Each word you read remains just long enough in your immediate memory to make the transition from one word or idea to the next. You discarded immediately many of the words you read, but you had to remember them long enough to make sense out of them.

The major problem with immediate memory is that it is extremely limited. That is, we are able to respond to only one thing at a time, and the amount of information we can retain is limited to approximately two to four items. Another problem with immediate memory is that it requires singular attention to determine which items require prompt response and which items require transfer from the immediate memory before they decay and are lost forever.

Short-term memory comes into play after the information has been sorted out as being important enough to remember. It sometimes is called a "working memory" because it is the system we use to remember information that must be recalled or responded to within seconds or minutes after receiving it. Short-term memory is what we use to look up a telephone number and remember it only long enough to dial. The basic difference between short-term and immediate memory is that short-term memory allows us to remember several things at once, for periods of time greater than one second. One negative aspect of short-term memory is that it is a rather limited system, capable of remembering only a maximum of seven items at a time. The short-term memory also is subject to rapid information loss — although not as rapid as that of the immediate memory. Because disturbances can cause memory loss, the short-term memory can even be overloaded, causing us to forget "everything" taken in at the time of the overload. This is why reasonable study schedules and study breaks are encouraged.

Long-term memory is used for information that must be stored for long periods (days, months, years) before use. Retrieving information from the long-term memory collection requires a search. If the long-term memory is unorganized, a big load is placed on the short-term memory. For that reason it is important to process incoming information correctly or else it will be unretrievable. The major advantages of the long-term memory system are (1) its limitless capacity to store information and (2) the number of items it can retain. Long-term memory facilitates learning and memorization of new material, and it is believed that the more information in the long-term memory, the easier it is to enter new information (Cermak, 1975).

To store information in the long-term memory requires attention, organization, and association (Fig. 3–1). Attention can be defined as focusing on material we want to remember and the ability to block any disturbing stimuli. The primary purpose of attention is to determine what is important enough to remember. Organization is the art of putting memory in order. Imagine that your mind is an expanding library of all your previously acquired knowledge, stored by appropriate categories. Each time new knowledge is acquired, it is added to any associated facts that were previously stored, waiting to be checked out. If a particular category of facts is used or added to only infrequently, it is treated as inactive and displaced to make room for new or additional facts. This process is unfortunate because inactive information sometimes becomes difficult to locate or even may be lost.

One popular method of remembering things is called *association*, a technique that involves forming an association with a fact. Engaging in this activity leads you to learn and think more about that fact, with a result that the more facts you associate with an item of memory, the more permanently those facts will be stored.

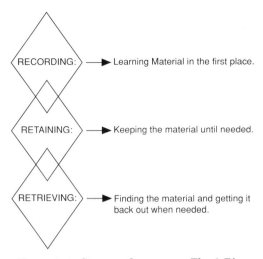

Figure 3–1. Stages of memory: The 3 R's.

Inaccurate memory. Humans have a tendency to alter and distort details. This tendency often occurs when some parts of a memory fail to fade in a uniform manner and are held together, but with missing or altered details. The motivation to distort the reality of events and experiences can be traced to our desire to make memories what we wish were so. By doing so, we support our beliefs and values, as well as our notions and hopes, and are able to defend our prejudices. Often we add details to our recollection of events to complete and make sense out of sketchy or incomplete memories. By filling in and rounding out missing details, we can create a memory that is satisfyingly whole or complete.

Although it is impossible to eliminate inaccurate remembering altogether, it is possible to decrease it to some extent. The key lies in remembering well and correctly. You can guard against inaccuracies by taking notes to ensure the precise remembrance of the information you want to recall. If you understand a subject clearly from the start, errors in thinking are not likely to occur. Your memory also improves if you prepare your body for the task. By resting and getting sufficient sleep and by healthy eating habits (particularly eating breakfast), your brain's ability to function is improved.

Forgetting. If you have ever failed to recall a name or a fact for a test, you understand the frustration of forgetting. Imagine, however, what would happen if you were unable to forget: the constant remembrance of pain, disappointment, and trauma would make life intolerable. Forgetting is a critical survival mechanism that allows the memory of painful experiences to lessen somewhat in intensity and eventually to fade. We have learned that high pleasure and pain levels enhance remembering, making it possible to retain painful physical or emotional memories and to remember them as needed. It is when the rewards of remembering do not reach such highs that we have a tendency to forget. This characteristic explains the common failure to remember names, dates, places, and material we do not understand, and it illustrates why it is important to make what you want to learn interesting; otherwise you must find artificial ways of remembering factual data.

Memorization. Memories can be stimulated in both a conscious and a subconscious fashion. Health care professionals often relate how the sensory triggers of sight, sound, touch, and smell frequently are associated with a particular patient or disease. Although these factors were not intentionally memorized, they still were registered in a subconscious fashion.

Conscious or intentional memorization occurs only when we deliberately and systematically devise ways to recall specific facts. As such it relies heavily on both perception and attention.

Our perceptions are greatly influenced by previous memories; therefore, possessing a memory bank rich in similar information increases the accuracy of our perceptions. The mind is not only a computer-like processor of information; it also is a museum that stores experiences and images. Thus, when sonographers scan patients, the brief appearance of a partial shape or prominent echo-pattern often is sufficient to trigger recognition. Experience has shown that any increase in such memories is proportional to the sonographer's scanning activity. This occurrence can be explained by the fact that during a sonographic examination, each time information is displayed on the viewing monitor, it also is stored in the sonographer's memory. In addition, it has been demonstrated that sonographers who have logged many transducer hours reproduce their perceptions of patients' anatomy more rapidly and with greater detail and accuracy than do novice sonographers. The veteran sonographers subconsciously demonstrate their ability to retrieve data from a large body of organized and synthesized information.

As stated previously, attention requires concentration and a sharp focus on a specific fact or activity, whereas concentration requires discipline and vigilance to ignore interfering thoughts or distractions. By preparing yourself to receive new information and to learn

1. Baby's block bearing the letters A and C.
2. A "plus" sign.
3. A bowl of soup.
4. An "equal" sign.
5. Alphabet Soup

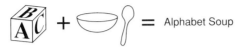

Figure 3–2. Visual associations.

something about a subject in advance, you can help improve your ability to concentrate.

Memory techniques. Whenever we are confronted with a large volume of new or unfamiliar information, or an inadequate amount of time in which to learn that information, it is common to use memory aids. The memory techniques most commonly employed are *clustering, relating, imagining,* and *mnemonics.*

Clustering is a method of memorizing long series of data by arranging them in segments. It usually is easier to remember numbers that are grouped in segments of three to five. This is how you recall your telephone number, your social security number, and your zip code.

Rhyming also can make remembering easier. When facts or phrases are set to music, they are easier to recall. Remember the songs you used for mastering the alphabet—*ABCD-EFG-HIJK-LMNOP*—and the rhyme you used for learning your numbers, *one, two, buckle my shoe?*

The use of visual or verbal associations also enhance remembering by bridging memory gaps, and some examples of association are shown in Figure 3–2. The most successful associations are tied to prior knowledge. For instance, you might choose to remember the number of white and black keys on a piano (52 white keys and 36 black keys) by associating them to the facts that there are *52* weeks in a year and *36* inches in a yard. Sometimes it is the similarities in spelling two different words that can cause memory difficulties, for example, the words *stationery* and *stationary.* In this instance it might be helpful to remember that the *e* in stationery stands for *letters.*

The use of acronyms and acrostics can make material meaningful by gathering information into clusters so that you do not have as much to remember. For example, the names of the Great Lakes form the acronym HOMES, which stands for *H*uron, *O*ntario, *M*ichigan, *E*rie, and *S*uperior. Acronyms also are widely used to represent associations, organizations, government agencies, and military titles and terms (Table 3–1).

Another popular mnemonic technique involves creating a rhyme or a story that contains the facts to be remembered. To remind us when to begin and end the use of daylight savings time, we use the following saying:

> *Spring ahead* in the spring,
> *Fall back* in the fall.

Medical students traditionally have used an acrostic to remember the twelve cranial nerves (olfactory, optic, oculomotor, trochlear, trigeminal, abducens, facial, auditory vestibular, glossopharyngeal, vagus, spinal accessory, hypoglossal) by assigning the first letter of each nerve to a word in a sentence:

> *O*n *O*ld *O*lympus' *T*owering *T*op *A* *F*at *A*rmed *G*erman *V*iewed *S*ome *H*ops.

First-letter mnemonics provide dual cues to help retrieve items and also tell us how many items are to be remembered, so that we know when they have all been recalled.

The memory technique that works best for concrete objects and actions, such as remembering the items on our shopping lists, is imagery, or visualization. The major drawback to this technique is that it works poorly on abstract concepts (such as justice and mercy). Whenever ultrasonic equipment controls are mentioned, most sonographers mentally visualize an instrument console and each control that is being discussed. Hearing a sonography term such as *increased gain* might trigger the memory of an ultrasound scan filled with predominantly bright echoes.

The obvious value of memory aids is that they make us organize, associate, and visualize meaningful information, forcing us to

---

Table 3–1. Acronyms as Memory Aids

COMMON ACRONYMS

SDMS	Society of Diagnostic Medical Sonographers
UN	United Nations
NCO	Noncommissioned officer
SNAFU	Situation normal, all fouled up!

concentrate—to pay attention. What seldom is mentioned is the painful fact that *what you understand,* does not require memorization. It is *what you do not understand* that you memorize.

Deductive Reasoning

One of the greatest challenges in teaching sonography lies in getting students who are the product of American schools to develop the skill of deductive reasoning. This form of thinking involves drawing conclusions from facts and depends not only on the storage of facts in our memory bank but on the ability to recover and to logically manipulate that information to correlate with the clinical questions at hand. Logic represents an important creative thinking tool that will be especially useful in the practical phases of the creative thinking process, when you are evaluating ideas and preparing them for action.

Effective Listening

If you wish to learn, it is imperative that you increase your reading rate and listening skills. Studies have shown that people rarely listen with maximum efficiency, and they consciously pay attention to only 25 percent of what they hear. The average speaking rate has been measured at approximately 100 words per minute, whereas the average listening and thinking rate takes place at 400 to 500 words per minute (McKeachie, 1978). Such a great time lag encourages the mind to wander. Knowing this fact should prompt you to develop methods to increase your attention span by becoming an effective listener.

Most of the time we listen inefficiently. Maidment has estimated that three fourths of each workday is spent talking and listening, and three fourths of what we do hear is heard imprecisely. The regret is that three fourths of what we hear accurately we forget within three weeks (Maidment, 1984). Although listening is the most often used communicative skill, it is the one in which we have been given the least training. This presents a serious problem, because the end product of listening is *knowing.*

Listening involves sensing, and it goes beyond hearing or assessing only the spoken words. Good listeners think more broadly as a result of hearing and understanding more facts and points of view. Because listeners look at problems with fresh eyes, they combine what they learn in more unlikely ways and are apt to develop new and valuable ideas. If given a choice, effective listeners will focus on ideas inasmuch as facts can be resurrected later.

Two important mental functions in effective listening are *recall* and *comprehension*. Recall is a *have-or-have-not* function involving memory. It is that portion of what we hear that can be restated later. In contrast, comprehension is a *have-to-have* function involving mastery, or that portion of what we hear that is thoroughly understood and intelligently applied. A special kind of listening occurs when we are silent, attentive, and receptive. This *third ear* mulls over, interprets, speculates, posits, and reviews incoming information (Maidment, 1984).

To be an effective listener you must be motivated. In other words, you must have an interest in or reason for listening to what is being said. Effective listeners listen without prejudice to avoid ignoring or filtering out details or tuning out any speakers who do not match their own ideas or values.

If you want to get the most out of the information dispensed during classroom lectures, it is important that you come to class prepared to listen. If you have completed all of your lesson assignments, you will be able to put everything else out of your mind and to concentrate on the subject being discussed. You should also view classroom lectures as give-and-take sessions between the instructor and the students and use class discussion as a means of getting the facts straight or asking for explanations of any puzzling concepts.

Effective Note-Taking

Because it is impossible to remember everything that is said in a lecture, it is critical to jot down *only* the *important* facts. Because writing is time-consuming, note-taking should be limited to key words or phrases to serve as reminders. After the lecture you can review your notes and fill in the missing parts.

By organizing in outline form the material covered in the lecture, you can develop your own personal study aid. Make notes of the topics and the major points under each one. Recognize the importance of any phrases that an instructor repeats or writes on the chalkboard or overhead projector, and underline them in your notes. Train yourself to take down the *sense* of what an instructor is saying rather than try to include every word. Place question marks near anything that is unclear, and ask about it later. If necessary, rewrite your notes to help establish the information more firmly in your mind. Your notes should help you review a subject and provide correct and complete information. Flash cards, based on your notes and arranged in a logical order, provide another highly effective method to test your understanding of a subject.

Skillful Reading

Reading to comprehend is a complex and intellectual activity that can be achieved only through anticipation and evaluation of the material. Although speed-reading techniques may enable you to "read" large volumes of material, such techniques are worthless if comprehension is sacrificed.

A simple way to remember the main steps in effectively studying a reading assignment based on the work of E. L. Thomas and H. A. Robinson uses the acronym *PQRST* to remind students how to maximize their studies (Thomas and Robinson, 1982).

The PQRST method

P: Preview. Scan the material first by looking at the images and reading the captions and charts. Read all of the material in the titles and subtitles of the chapter and all of the words in italics. Read any available summaries or objectives. Scanning will enable you to identify the main thought or general idea. If there is an accompanying workbook, *read* the questions.

Q: Question. Ask yourself what the chapter is about and what major points it makes. Ask what the objectives of reading the chapter are so you know what is expected of you. Try to answer the questions in any workbook or manual that might accompany the text.

R: Reread/review. Read the chapter carefully as many times as necessary to understand the material. It may be helpful to read only one page at a time and then recall as much of the material as you can. Performing the recall aloud will use two senses instead of only one and will enhance your memory. Review the important points, evaluating what you have read by relating it to your existing knowledge. Take notes if necessary.

S: State. State verbally, or in writing, the major points covered in the chapter. This process will clarify your understanding of the material if you explain it in your own words — preferably to another student, if possible.

T: Test. Test yourself. Read the chapter objectives, and see if you can perform all the skills without consulting the chapter. Answer any questions, and do the activities listed in any course workbook. Once you have successfully completed each of these steps, you should be ready for a mastery test of the material.

Reading technical materials

Different methods are required for reading technical material than for recreational reading. Looking up and learning new terms requires more time, as does taking notes of important points. By following the PQRST system already described, you can enhance your learning ability. If you repeat those steps until you understand the subject and space them over several days, you will be able to retain the material in both your short- and long-term memory.

To firmly fix information in your mind, you should make notes while you read, and take advantage of using several senses to reinforce your memory. The most logical way is to create an outline with main headings and notations under each heading. Try to put the main ideas (except for definitions) in your own words.

Your instructors will often assign *outside* reading of other books, pamphlets, and journal articles to add to your knowledge. The importance of becoming familiar with your institution's medical library cannot be overemphasized. Even after completion of your sonography program you should set aside time each month for routinely reviewing periodicals and new books on sonography or related subjects.

Presenting Material

If you are asked to give a journal review, the following suggestions definitely will make your task easier and allow you to maximize your own learning:

1. List the topic heading, and under it list the main points (use the subheadings of the article) and provide enough information to explain each point adequately.
2. Record the title and page for future reference (index cards are useful for filing, easy retrieval, or rearrangement).
3. Include any additional information that you may have found in other references.
4. Make a note of any information that puzzles you, to remind you to discuss it in class or to look it up in another reference source before your presentation.
5. Look up any unfamiliar words in the dictionary. Make a list or a set of flashcards of such words and their definitions, and use it as a quiz.
6. Work with a friend if the topic is a lengthy subject. In this way you can cover the material from a different perspective – keeping the audience interested – and rehearse by testing each other's presentations.

If you are asked to make a case presentation, it is important to review all available clinical information and to add to it any relevant information derived from current resources, such as journal articles. Table 3–2 lists the components of a case study or review and suggestions on its presentation.

Table 3–2. Case Review

Components

Case history

Requisition

Sonography data

Official report

Follow-up

Pathology review

Case history

Include patient's age, sex, symptoms, referral route, physical and
laboratory findings.

Requisition

Note clinical question(s), type of sonography study requested, referring
physician's clinical comments.

Sonography data

Arrange images in order in which they were obtained during examination.
Demonstrate normal structures first, then discuss abnormal structures
or disease. Include the sonographer's impressions regarding size,
location, consistency, and so forth.

Official report

Include the final report, and compare or contrast it with the sonographer's
impressions.

Follow-up

Note sequelae of any sort; surgical and/or pathology reports; any
additional diagnostic test results.

Pathology review

Discuss the prevalence of abnormal pathologic findings and report on any
supporting journal articles. Describe those clinical symptoms of the
patient that were representative and whether or not the scans obtained
were sufficient and representative.

Learning Aids

Many tools are available to aid sonography students in learning the complexities of diagnostic medical sonography. Films and video-tapes often are more valuable than written materials because they demonstrate action. Along with slides, they also may demonstrate rare diseases unlikely to be encountered in the normal course of a training program. To obtain maximum benefits, however, it is essential that you *know what to look for* in any film or tape, *before you view it.*

Field Trips

You can often get clearer impressions by observing rather than just reading about a subject or activity. To make the most of any field trip, you should learn in advance about the place you are visiting and what to look for once you are there. Afterward, you and your fellow students should be prepared to discuss what you have seen.

Teaching Machines

Students who have been out of school for a few years often feel overwhelmed by the large amount and variety of educational hardware available in sonography programs. Calculators, computer terminals, software, and measuring devices are all learning aids that should be fairly easy to operate and use if you take the time to become familiar with the concept as well as the equipment.

Role Playing

For students inexperienced in actually working with patients and interacting with medical personnel, role playing is one of the best available methods for gaining confidence (Lea, 1983). Sonographers are expected to maintain a comfortable flow of conversation with patients before, throughout, and after completion of all examinations. They also are required to communicate skillfully with physicians and other health professionals. When students act the roles of patient, sonographer, and physician, they often discover different approaches and solutions to common sonography problems. Role playing also can prepare you to better understand your patients by tuning in to nonverbal gestures, subtle meanings, inner feelings, and unstated messages.

Effective Studying

Studying is much easier and more effective if it is planned. If you have been out of school for some time and are no longer in the habit of studying, establishing good study habits may be difficult at first. Study periods should be scheduled when you are most alert and attentive, and your study environment should be arranged so that distractions are reduced. Finding a quiet place to study at home—away from other residents—should be a priority. Ideally, a suitable place should be well-lighted, with sufficient space for writing and spreading books out conveniently. It also should be quiet enough to avoid distractions or interruptions. Assemble everything you need before you begin to study. Keep your work area neat, and provide yourself simple comforts such as a straight-backed chair and a cool room to help you concentrate and stay alert. Compose a study plan to avoid wasting time. Also, finish one project before starting another. It is difficult to concentrate if you skip from subject to subject while studying. Most important of all, take a "break" every now and then. Remember, the mind can absorb only what the posterior can endure!

TESTS AND EVALUATIONS

You must become accustomed to taking examinations or tests, because they provide a method to evaluate progress and to prepare students for registry or certifying examinations after graduation. Much of our educational system has taught us to look for "the one right answer." This approach is fine for some situations, but too many of us have the tendency to stop looking after the *first* answer has been found. The following material describes the various types of tests used in sonography programs.

Objective Tests

The most commonly used tests are written tests, which are answered by selecting a correct response from a group of alternatives or by filling in spaces. Objective tests can be presented in the formats that follow.

Multiple choice. Questions are situational in nature, and usually only one answer is correct. Some multiple choice tests, however, are constructed so that several answers may be correct. You are then expected to choose the *best* answer from a list of several options. Determine which approach is expected.

True-false. You are given a statement to evaluate and must decide whether it is right or wrong.

Completion. Missing words or phrases are included in a sentence. You must complete the sentence to make it true.

Matching. Two columns of words or phrases are provided, and you are asked to match each item in the first column with the related item in the second column. Check to see if the number of answers equals the number of questions or if there are more answers than questions. Determine whether answers may be used more than once.

Subjective Tests

The most common form of subjective test is the essay test. You may be asked (1) to define or explain a term or concept or (2) to describe how you would handle a given situation or solve a specific problem. Plan your answers before you write, and remember to express your ideas clearly and briefly. You may find an outline format particularly effective in writing your reply.

Test-Taking Skills

There are many tips and tricks to improving test performance, but undoubtedly the most important of them all is to *read the instructions!* Once you have finished reading the instructions, it is recommended that you follow this routine:

1. Go through the examination once, and answer all the items about which you are fairly certain. This exercise may possibly provide answers to earlier questions that seemed difficult.
2. Go through the examination again, and answer any questions that are now obvious to you.
3. For any remaining unanswered multiple choice questions, try to eliminate the obviously incorrect responses. Then choose the answer you first thought was right. If you are totally stumped, answer "B" or "2" has been statistically shown to be the right answer. Teachers are reluctant to place the correct answer in either first or last position; instead they place it in the middle of seductive alternatives.
4. Once you have answered all test questions, it is a good idea to go through the whole test once again and check your choices to make sure that they are the ones you still regard as correct and that you have made no clerical errors—especially if recording them on separate answer sheets.

Testing Equipment

Machine scoring requires the use of a preprinted answer sheet. There usually are from three to six answer slots for each question. Be sure to read and follow the test instructions carefully. Check that the answer you selected is matched correctly to the appropriate question. Also be aware that machine malfunctions can occur, causing your answer sheet to be incorrectly marked.

Computerized testing

You may be asked to use a computer terminal to take a test. In such tests you usually receive immediate feedback on whether your answer was right or wrong. If wrong, you probably will be told the correct answer.

TRANSITION FROM CLASSROOM
TO CLINICAL SETTING

Clinical training and experience are among the most variable aspects of sonography programs in the United States. The design and implementation of your clinical activities will be heavily governed by institutional regulations developed in response to legal, ethical, governmental, and financial pressures.

Scanning Arts

Ideally, you should be provided with firsthand experience not only in the observation of but in the manipulation of sonography equipment on a living patient. If regulations prohibit the use of live models or patients for scanning instruction, the use of scanning objects and "phantoms" may be substituted. You must practice until you have developed the requisite complex scanning skills, based on eye-hand coordination, and have become familiar and proficient in using the equipment to make anatomic measurements.

Individual instruction is the exception rather than the rule in most sonography programs. However, a reasonable instructor-to-student ratio, as well as a reasonable student-to-machine ratio, should be in place. Learning to operate ultrasound equipment and to scan patients is no different from other eye-hand coordinated activities, such as learning to play the piano or playing tennis or golf. Some group instruction is acceptable, but until you are able to relate "one-on-one," there is little hope of mastering the art and science of medical sonography. Although films and demonstrations are important, they are definitely secondary to sensorimotor activities.

Scanning laboratories

Your first rotation from the classroom may be to the sheltered environment of a *scanning-arts laboratory.* Here you will have the opportunity to integrate your classroom knowledge of the physical principles of ultrasound by using various types of ultrasound instrumentation. Scanning test objects or "volunteers," or both, will give you hands-on experience in setting up an ultrasound unit, manipulating the transducer, positioning patients, making measurements of specified anatomic structures, and using various recording devices. As you actually perform the scanning protocols you have been studying, you will begin to appreciate how sonographers are required to tailor every examination to meet the needs of patients' individual body types. Through trial and error—but with the helpful direction of your clinical instructor—you should develop familiarity and confidence in scanning techniques before moving on to working with actual patients.

Clinical instructors often use the time in the practice laboratory for role-playing sessions to develop the ability to converse with future patients, to answer their questions, to explain their own procedures, and to learn how to listen effectively. Having the chance to practice in a stress-free environment will provide a solid base for launching your clinical skills.

Clinical Observation and Assistance

The next step may be a familiarization visit to a clinical site to observe day-to-day operations. While there, you may be asked to assist staff members by carrying out ancillary tasks such as helping the patients onto the scanning table or recording measurements and images as the sonographer directs. Once you are able to perform these tasks correctly, you can progress to the more independent phases of performing all aspects of the ultrasound examination under the direct supervision of either your clinical instructor or another registered sonographer.

As you make the classroom-to-clinical transition, your competence in meeting the educational objectives of your program will be evaluated. Remember that competency levels vary from student to student, so that comparing yourself or competing with other students is unrealistic. Instead, set your sights on performing better tomorrow than you did today.

Performance Evaluations

Although the field of sonography has not yet reached uniform agreement on every aspect of clinical performance (Lea, 1981), preliminary recommendations have been drawn up both by the SDMS and by the AIUM, and your program may have adopted one of them. Student sonographers should understand *what* is going to be evaluated, *how often* evaluations will take place, and *what type* of evaluation instrument will be used.

Most evaluations are divided into two categories: product and process competencies. Product competencies relate to the skills necessary to perform specialty sonographic examinations; they cover a wide range of activities—from obtaining patient history to reviewing the sonographic images with the sonologist. Process competencies are universal skills—such as motivation, appearance, and patient interaction—that transcend the various ultrasound specialties.

Student sonographers must become familiar with what is clinically expected of them if they are to successfully complete the practical portions of their training. Table 3–3 gives examples of the components of typical sonography evaluation instruments. To avoid anxiety and fear, sonographers should be informed as to *when* evaluations will take place and whether the evaluation will be used for instruction or for grading purposes. In either case the instructor should review the evaluation with you, point by point, as soon as possible (while memory of the activity is still fresh) to obtain feedback and to provide reinforcement. If you fail any of the program's goals and objectives, you should be given additional instruction and assignments and the opportunity to perform for reevaluation.

Often students are unaware that they have the right to evaluate their sonography programs and to make suggestions and recommendations for improvement (Table 3–4).

Clinical Competency

A competent sonographer must possess many diverse skills. The following list describes the minimum requirements of general proficiency:

1. Extensive knowledge of the physical principles of diagnostic ultrasound to ensure the ability to recognize and overcome any scanning difficulties that may arise during an examination.
2. A working knowledge of the mechanics and operational features of many types of ultrasound systems—necessary because of the broad-based nature of medical sonography.
3. In-depth appreciation of pathology and pathophysiology, as well as the anatomy and physiology of pertinent body systems. Only with this type of educational foundation can sonographers develop the ability to tailor or redirect an ultrasound study to each patient's body habitus and disease process.
4. The ability to survey and scan clinically relevant areas, correlating clinical information with sonographic findings.
5. Recognition and recording of representative images and measurements of both normal and abnormal findings. Recognition of any indications that a more detailed examination is needed.

Table 3–3. Components of a Competency Evaluation

Element	Behavioral Indications
PROCESS	
Appearance	Hygiene Adherence to dress code
Dependability	Punctuality
Organization	Attention to detail
Patient interaction	Attitude Communication Knowledge of basic patient care
Adaptability	Cooperation Acceptance of criticism
Initiative	Self-confidence Self-actualizing Intellectually curious Interest in continuing education
Judgment	Ability to remain within the limits of competency
PRODUCT	
Preliminary	Patient greeting/identification Obtaining patient history Patient positioning Equipment selection Selection of proper scanning protocol
Performance	Ability to select and adequately scan and measure specific areas of interest Ability to reevaluate patient positioning, need for additional scans Documentation of diagnostic images Pleasant and informative interaction with patient during performance of examination
Completion	Written and oral responses to supervising physician regarding scans Reassurance and dismissal of patient Documentation of examination and results in appropriate logs, teaching files, and so on Cleaning and preparation of work area for next examination

Table 3–4. Legitimate Topics for Student Evaluation of Program and Courses

Classroom and clinical experience	Academic and clinical instructors
Academic and clinical instruction	Program director
Clinical rotation	Medical director
Courses: most/least useful	Sonography program

6. Evaluation of patients' clinical and laboratory histories in order to scan the proper anatomic areas and to know which images to record (those that demonstrate or rule out the clinical problem) for the sonologist's review.
7. Familiarity with the differential diagnoses of common diseases in the patient population.
8. The ability to function as part of the diagnostic team by becoming an assistant to or a resource for the physician.
9. The ability to discuss procedures with the sonologist, referring physicians, and patients, as directed.
10. The capability to assume the role of teacher to students, staff members, and patients.
11. Willingness to engage in continuing education activities to ensure that proficiency is maintained.

EDUCATIONAL CURRICULA

Because of the multidisciplinary and dynamic nature of diagnostic medical sonography, it is crucial that students acquire not only the theory of the physical and applied principles but also clinical knowledge and the skills that will permit them to achieve specialty performance objectives and perform at the level of responsibility expected of sonographers.

Table 3–5 outlines a minimum curriculum for a one-year course of study in diagnostic medical sonography. These suggestions may be expanded, depending on the institutional setting of the sonography program.

Programs of Study

There are currently several educational pathways to becoming a registered diagnostic medical sonographer (RDMS). Various types of

Table 3–5. Curriculum for One-Year Course of Study

I. PHYSICAL SCIENCES
  A. Survey of acoustic physics
   1. Knowledge and understanding of the physical sciences on which the concepts of diagnostic ultrasound are based
   2. Basic principles of high-frequency sound production and propagation
  B. Medical applications of ultrasound
   1. Overview of therapeutic ultrasound
   2. Basic concepts of diagnostic ultrasound
    a. characteristics of sound/tissue interaction
    b. biologic effects of diagnostic ultrasound
    c. instrumentation: modalities, signal processing, and calibration
    d. clinical applications and related instrumentation

II. APPLIED BIOLOGIC SCIENCES
  A. Human structure and function: Emphasis on organ/system relationships
  B. Physiology and cross-sectional anatomy: Emphasis on scanning planes
  C. Pathophysiology
  D. Histopathology and acoustic properties

III. CLINICAL MEDICINE
  A. Diagnosis of the pathology and pathophysiology of sonographically visible organs/systems
   1. Historical/clinical findings
   2. Differential diagnosis
  B. Sonographic procedures relevant to clinical evaluation of disease
  C. Related diagnostic procedures and their limitations
   1. imaging
   2. laboratory
   3. funtional

IV. SONOGRAPHY
  A. Scanning protocols
  B. Scanning techniques
  C. Quality control
  D. Interpretation

V. PATIENT CARE
  A. Health care delivery
  B. Patient evaluation/psychology
  C. Emergency care
  D. Medicolegal aspects
  E. Medical ethics

Table 3–5. Curriculum for One-Year Course of Study
Continued

VI. ADMINISTRATION
   A. Development of an ultrasound
      facility
      1. Design
      2. Equipment selection
   B. Operation of an ultrasound
      facility
      1. Scheduling
      2. Record keeping
      3. Supplies
      4. Fiscal management principles
      5. Departmental and interdepartmental
      relations
      6. Personnel management/
      procedures

sonography programs exist in this country. Some are formal educational programs and may be accredited; others are short-term, informal programs that provide limited education and focus on basic skills training. The latter type of program assumes that students will return to the workplace and continue their studies and training independently, but under the direction of their supervising physician. The availability of such options makes it important to distinguish the difference between *education* and *training*.

Education involves the process of systematically developing and cultivating knowledge, the mind, character, and skills through formal schooling, teaching, and instruction. In contrast, training is the systematic, practical instruction and drill in a subject that guides, conditions, or controls certain actions to bring about a desired condition. Before selecting a course of study it is important to evaluate whether you will receive only (1) education, (2) only training, or (3) both education and training.

Three types of formal educational programs currently exist in the United States: hospital-based programs (1 year), community college programs (1 to 2 years), and baccalaureate degree programs (4 years).

Long-term training programs. Hospital-based programs were among the first formal programs offered to train sonographers. A diploma or certificate usually is granted upon satisfactory course completion. Classroom activities often are limited to the appropriate sciences and usually are conducted on site, along with clinical rotations. The emphasis of the hospital-based program is on clinical performance.

In community college associate-degree programs and university-based baccalaureate programs, greater emphasis is placed on theory. Classes usually consist of nonscientific as well as basic science courses. The didactic sessions generally are held on campus, with clinical rotations taking place in area hospitals or clinics. The educational focus of these institutions is to provide a *well-rounded educational experience* that may serve as a springboard to advanced studies and employment in managerial or instructional positions.

Short-term training programs. These programs usually vary in length from one week to three months. They generally are proprietary programs that offer limited courses intended to familiarize the attendees with the operation and potential clinical usefulness of diagnostic ultrasound systems. This type of course requires its students to continue their training through self-study and supervised scanning in the workplace.

On-the-job training. In some remote settings, on-the-job training is the only available training option to providing a diagnostic ultrasound service for the community. Supplementary instructional videotapes, correspondence courses, and occasional visits by the manufacturers' application specialists are valuable resources.

SUMMARY

Humans are capable of three types of memory: immediate, short-term, and long-term. None of these memory systems operates totally independent of the other; that is, long-term memory depends on short-term memory, and short-term memory is dependent on immediate memory. Memory is improved when we (1) learn and organize new facts and (2) systematically relate them to our previously acquired knowledge.

Proper storage of information is the key to its retrieval. Experience has shown that the following steps must be followed to remember useful information:

- *Consciously decide* — to remember it
- *Repeat it* — to help fix its meaning
- *Refresh or review it* — at intervals
- *Understand it* — by searching for meaning

Artificial memory aids have been used for years and are widely accepted in learning certain types of material. However, the range of items that can be committed to memory in this fashion is quite limited. For the majority of learning situations it is best (1) to deliberately intend to remember, (2) to actively use as many senses as possible, and (3) to refresh your memory often.

In the education and training of sonographers it is necessary to test not only students' comprehension of the material that has been presented but also their skills in manipulating the transducer on an endless variety of anatomically variable patients.

The final form of testing employs clinical evaluations that are based on such factors as performance, attitude, interpersonal relations, reactions to criticism, efforts to improve, appearance, health habits, punctuality, dependability, ethics, and day-to-day responses in the classroom.

Several types of educational and training opportunities are available to sonographers in the United States. *Formal training* can be acquired in hospitals, community colleges, and universities. *Informal training* is available through short-term programs (proprietary or nonproprietary), commercially sponsored customer courses, and on-the-job training.

Supply and demand currently play pivotal roles in the education and employment of sonographers. It is assumed that informal, short-term education eventually will be phased out of existence if, and when, formal programs adequately meet the personal needs of diagnostic medical sonography.

REFERENCES

Cermak, L.: Improving Your Memory. New York: McGraw-Hill, 1975.

Lea, J. H.: Developing competency-based clinical education in sonography. Medical Ultrasound 1981; 5(1):1-4.

Lea, J. H.: The value of role playing in sonography education. Medical Ultrasound 1983; 7(2):81-82.

Maidment, R.: Tuning In. A Guide to Effective Listening. Gretna, La.: Pelican Publishing Co., 1984.

McKeachie, W. J.: Teaching Tips. A Guidebook for the Beginning College Teacher, 7th ed. Lexington, Mass.: D. C. Heath & Co., 1978.

Thomas, E. L., and Robinson, H. A.: Improving Reading in Every Class. Boston, Mass.: Allyn and Bacon, 1982.

▼

UNIT 4

Patient-Sonographer
Interaction

PART I
Basic Medical Techniques and Patient Care

LEARNING OBJECTIVES

Students who successfully complete Part I will be able to:

- Understand the obligations of the sonographer to patients, institution, and self.
- Explain the Patient's Bill of Rights.
- Describe patient reactions to illness.
- Understand how to measure vital signs.
- Discuss the safety considerations associated with patient care.
- List the components of good body mechanics.
- Describe the correct patient-transfer methods.
- Discuss the care of patients with tubes or tubings.
- Describe the sonographer's role in emergency medical situations.
- Discuss the sonographer's role in infection control.
- Discuss the impact of cultural beliefs on diagnosis and treatment.

As a sonographer you will work under the direction of a physician-sonologist to obtain diagnostic images of the patients entrusted to your care. Your training will teach you how to operate ultrasound instruments and to decipher echo information returning from the patient's body. You also should receive information on how to provide basic care to your patients.

Sonographer Obligations

To fulfill your role as a sonographer, you must be responsible to yourself, to your department or institution, and to your patients. From a physical standpoint you should be adequately rested and relaxed, practice good nutrition, and engage in exercise to promote your physical health. Maintaining good mental health also is important and requires that you recognize your own needs, strengths, and limitations. You must recognize any anxiety or distress you feel about any work-related situations that might interfere with your job performance. Leaving personal or family problems at home is just as important as leaving work problems at work. If you are unable to resolve problems in either area, you should seek proper counseling. Because caring for patients can be emotionally draining, you should have a means of rejuvenating yourself through physical exercise and enjoyable hobbies.

Developing a good self-image and viewing problems as challenges or opportunities rather than stumbling blocks will make it easier for you to accept criticism as a learning opportunity and not as a defeat. What will result is a sense of pride in your work and an eagerness to start each day.

Patient Rights

In addition to having the necessary knowledge and skills to perform competent sonographic examinations, you are responsible for the type of care you give your patients (Table 4–1).

All patients deserve to be treated with respect, dignity, and kindness. Remember that patients' needs come first, and learn to control any anger or frustration that might develop when you work with patients. You are expected to discuss matters pertinent to your patients *only* with authorized hospital personnel, not with your family and friends.

You should understand that patients have the right to information concerning their health care and to decision-making regarding their diagnosis and treatment. In some instances, patients may refuse care or tests, which makes it important that you try tactfully to reason with them by explaining the nature of the examination as it relates to their problem or illness. If a patient continues to refuse an examination, you should encourage him or her to contact the physician for a fuller explanation. Be sure to

Table 4–1. A Patient's Bill of Rights

1. The patient has the right to considerate and respectful care.
2. The patient has the right to obtain from his physician complete current information concerning his diagnosis, treatment, and prognosis in terms the patient can be reasonably expected to understand. When it is not medically advisable to give such information to the patient, the information should be made available to an appropriate person in his behalf. He has the right to know by name, the physician responsible for coordinating his care.
3. The patient has the right to receive from his physician information necessary to give informed consent prior to the start of any procedure and/or treatment. Except in emergencies, such information for informed consent should include but not necessarily be limited to the specific procedure and/or treatment, the medically significant risks involved, and the probable duration of incapacitation. Where medically significant alternatives for care or treatment exist, or when the patient requests information concerning medical alternatives, the patient has the right to such information. The patient also has the right to know the name of the person responsible for the procedures and/or treatment.
4. The patient has the right to refuse treatment to the extent permitted by law, and to be informed of the medical consequences of his action.
5. The patient has the right to every consideration of his privacy concerning his own medical care program. Case discussion, consultation, examination, and treatment are confidential and should be conducted discreetly. Those not directly involved in his care must have the permission of the patient to be present.
6. The patient has the right to expect that all communications and records pertaining to his care should be treated as confidential.
7. The patient has the right to expect that, within its capacity, a hospital must make reasonable response to the request of a patient for services. The hospital must provide evaluation, service and/or referral as indicated by the urgency of the case. When medically permissible, a patient may be transferred to another facility only after he has received complete information and explanation concerning the needs for and alternatives to such a transfer. The institution to which the patient is to be transferred must first have accepted the patient for transfer.

Reprinted with permission of the American Hospital Association, copyright 1972.

Table continued on following page

Table 4–1. A Patient's Bill of Rights *Continued*

8. The patient has the right to obtain information as to any relationship of his hospital to other health care and educational institutions insofar as his care is concerned. The patient has the right to obtain information as to the existence of any professional relationships among individuals, by name, who are treating him.
9. The patient has the right to be advised if the hospital proposes to engage in or perform human experimentation affecting his care or treatment. The patient has the right to refuse to participate in such research projects.
10. The patient has the right to expect reasonable continuity of care. He has the right to know in advance what appointment times and physicians are available and where. The patient has the right to expect that the hospital will provide a mechanism whereby he is informed by his physician or a delegate of the physician of the patient's continuing health care requirements following discharge.
11. The patient has the right to examine and receive an explanation of his bill regardless of source of payment.
12. The patient has the right to know what hospital rules and regulations apply to his conduct as a patient.

provide reassurance that you will gladly reschedule the examination at a mutually convenient time if the patient decides to undergo the procedure.

Patients have a right to privacy and may request that students, other observers, medical personnel, and family leave the room during the sonography examination. If any patients elect to have friends or family members present during their examination, you should inform them of the hospital rules and any policies that govern such requests. Some sonographers say they feel uncomfortable having "outsiders" looking on while they are scanning, even though there may be no regulations prohibiting their presence. If this situation arises, you must give a truthful explanation to the patient if there is inadequate space for viewing or if the presence of observers hinders your concentration and abilities. Often such situations can be eased if sonographers explain that they need time alone with the patient to get them ready for the examination and to take a series of scans for evaluation purposes. In return for such cooperation, you could offer to call the observers into the examination room for their own "showing." By following these suggestions, the discovery of unexpected pathologic findings can be controlled without causing anxiety to patients or their support group.

Another patient right involves the expectation of pleasant physical and emotional surroundings where the person's comfort, safety, and respect as an individual are ensured.

Patient environment

One of the most important considerations in the design of an ultrasound facility should be the patient and the sonographer's physical surroundings. For safety and comfort the following features should be considered:

- Proper ventilation and comfortable temperature
- Adequate lighting
- Comfortable and safe furnishings
- Equipment in good working order
- Reasonable access to bathroom facilities
- A safe and private area for disrobing and storing personal articles

It usually is the sonographer's duty to keep the examining room and equipment neat and clean. Any nondisposable medical equipment used by the patient should be properly cleansed immediately after an examination and returned to its proper place. Sonographers should contact housekeeping personnel for immediate services in the event of accidental spills.

Emotional surroundings

An ultrasound facility should offer a climate in which the patient is treated as an individual. Staff members should introduce themselves to patients and explain what they will be doing for them. Patients should be oriented to any procedures such as filling out admission or consent forms. Patient privacy should be respected at all times, particularly during dressing and undressing, during performance of ultrasound scans, and during use of bathroom facilities. If patients require assistance at any of these times, the sonographer should provide it in a mature and completely professional manner.

Allow your patients to freely express their thoughts, opinions, or beliefs. Be a good listener and do not impose your own beliefs on the patient. In the event that the examination you perform reveals serious illness or the threat of imminent death, remember that patients may wish to engage in spiritual practices or rituals. Show respect for their wishes, and provide assistance or privacy as indicated.

PATIENT CARE

Patient Reactions to Illness

Becoming a sonographer places you in a position to see the changes that disease and disability cause in people. You should understand that change is a series of gains and losses and that disease and disability interrupt the natural balance of the body and thus produce stress. Such stress can cause emotional reactions in your patients. Among the key emotional reactions you may encounter are the following states.

Anger. Anger toward others may be expressed verbally or physically.

Anxiety. Feelings of apprehension may cause patients to be unwilling to adjust to their new situation and cry, fear being alone, or act suspicious, hostile, or withdrawn. Anxiety also can produce physical changes such as rapid pulse, increased blood pressure and respirations, headaches, nervousness, excessive perspiration, or rapid speech.

Frustration and helplessness. The longer it takes to diagnose and treat the illness, the more frustrated the patient will become. In our society, men are especially vulnerable to feelings of loss of control and independence because strength is a major asset in their self-image.

Grief. Grieving is the process of adjusting to the reality of a loss. Whether it is a loss of health or the loss of a pregnancy, your patients will be flooded with emotions. Shock, denial, anger, bargaining, guilt, and depression are common feelings that grieving patients must work through before they are able to accept their losses.

Guilt. Patients who feel that they are unable to perform their accustomed roles in life (such as mother or breadwinner) usually respond with anger (why me?) or view their loss as a punishment. Particularly in the area of loss resulting from pregnancy interruption, a woman tends to critically examine every aspect of her life to discover where she was at fault. The response to guilt can take many forms: withdrawal, blame, fault finding, or physical complaints.

Depression. Feelings of helplessness, sadness, or lack of vitality are characteristic of the depressed person. Severely depressed patients often complain of insomnia, early morning fatigue, loss of appetite, and numerous physical complaints.

Dependency. Some patients are highly demanding, whereas others show their dependency by an inability to follow directions or by attempting tasks beyond their capabilities.

Suspicion. Feelings of mistrust may overcome some patients, making them fearful and feeling that everyone and everything is against them. Often, the one-on-one environment of the sonography laboratory encourages patients to talk about their feelings. Although as a sonographer you are not responsible for evaluating and treating your patients' emotional reactions, you should share your observations and concerns with the referring physician or charge nurse. By all means, try to be a good listener.

If a patient responds negatively to being scanned and becomes upset, do not allow yourself to get upset as well. Try to be patient, understanding, and secure enough to let your patients know you care.

Vital Signs

The term *vital signs* refers to temperature, pulse, respirations, and blood pressure as indicators of the functioning of the body. During the course of a sonographic examination sonographers may be required to assess the pulse, respirations, and blood pressure as part of the scanning protocol. Careful, accurate measurement of each of these parameters is essential.

As a part of the assessment of vital signs you also should observe the patient's total condition: color, skin temperature, and any comments about how the patient feels and reacts. If you have never worked with patients before, the following review will establish guidelines for taking vital signs.

Pulse

The pulse is the beat of the heart that can be felt as a vibration within the walls of the arteries. With each heart beat, blood forced into the arteries causes them to swell or expand, producing arterial pulses that can be felt with your fingers.

The most convenient site for taking the pulse is the radial artery, located on the thumb side of the wrist. However, other arteries close to the skin also provide pulse sites (e.g., temporal, carotid, mandibular, femoral, popliteal).

Pulse *rate* refers to the number of beats per minute, whereas *rhythm* refers to the time interval between beats. You should evaluate whether there is a smooth and regular rhythm as opposed to irregular rhythms with skipped beats. The strength of a pulse refers to its force and usually is described as bounding or weak and thready.

Substances such as coffee, tea, tobacco, or certain drugs can cause rhythm irregularities. Shock and hemorrhage can cause a weak, thready pulse, whereas fever can produce a bounding pulse.

The normal adult pulse rate is 60 to 65 beats per minute (bpm). Newborn infants have a pulse rate of 120 to 140 bpm, whereas women, children, and elderly patients usually have a slightly faster than normal pulse rate. Athletes in good condition generally have a slower pulse — below 60 bpm (Rosdahl, 1985).

Abnormally rapid pulse rates (over 100 bpm) are termed *tachycardia*. Abnormally slow pulse rates (below 60 bpm) are termed *bradycardia*. Exercise, strong emotions, fever, pain, and shock can all elevate the pulse. In contrast, resting, depression, and certain drugs (such as digitalis) can lower the pulse.

The pulse is felt by gently compressing the artery over a bony prominence in the area. *Never feel the pulse with your own thumb,* because it has a pulse of its own that interferes with obtaining an accurate reading of the patient's pulse.

Obtaining an arterial pulse. Proceed as follows:

1. Explain to the patient what you plan to do.
2. Place the patient's arm in a comfortable, resting position.
3. Identify the location of the artery by placing your fingertips over the artery and pressing firmly enough to feel the pulsations (Fig. 4–1).
4. Count the beats of the pulse (starting the count with *zero*) for at least 30 seconds. Multiply this number by 2 to obtain the beats per minute.

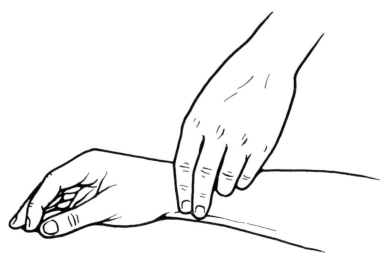

Figure 4–1. Taking a radial pulse. Support the patient's arm in a comfortable position, and never use the thumb to feel the patient's pulse.

5. If irregularities are noted (too fast/too slow), count the beats for a full minute and report your findings.

Respiration

The oxygen and carbon dioxide exchange that takes place in the lungs is referred to as *respiration*. The respiratory process begins with the delivery of oxygen to body cells via blood that has passed through the lungs. The cells give off accumulated carbon dioxide to the blood, which returns it to the lungs. There, the potentially dangerous carbon dioxide wastes are exhaled out of the body in the act of breathing (Burke, 1980).

Breathing can be defined as the expansion (inspiration) and contraction (respiration) of the lungs. Normal breathing is quiet, effortless, and regular in rhythm; it occurs at a rate of 16 to 20 breaths per minute in the normal adult.

Rate, rhythm, and the depth and character of the respirations should be noted. The *rate* refers to the number of respirations per minute. *Rhythm* refers to the regular rate of breathing and a symmetric movement of the chest. *Depth* refers to the amount of air taken in with each respiration (normal, shallow, deep). *Character* refers to the quality of respirations (e.g., quiet, wheezing, coughing).

Any injuries to the lungs, chest muscles, or diaphragm will affect breathing. It also is important to note any positions the patient may need to assume to breathe easily — sitting up or standing as opposed to lying down. Also note any difficulty in breathing (dyspnea) or changes in the patient's color (cyanosis or pallor).

Counting respirations. Respirations are counted as follows:

1. Count the respirations without the patient being aware of what you are doing. Watch the patient's breathing, and count a breathing sequence (in and out) as one respiration.
2. Start the count at zero, and continue counting respirations for at least 30 seconds. Multiply the number by 2 to arrive at the respirations per minute.
3. If irregularities are observed (rate, rhythm, patient appearance, or behavior), count the respirations for one full minute and report your findings.

Blood pressure

Blood pressure is the pressure of circulating blood against arterial walls that is produced by the pumping action of the heart. The pressure of blood within the arteries is highest whenever the heart contracts, and this pressure is called the *systolic* pressure. Between beats, when the heart rests, arterial pressure is at its lowest and is called *diastolic* pressure.

Heart activity can be heard as "thumping" sounds in the large arteries of the limbs. These sounds can be translated into numbers representing millimeters of mercury (mm Hg) on a manometer. When taking a blood pressure reading, you will be listening with a stethoscope and watching the numbers on a manometer.

The normal adult blood pressure is about 120/80 (120 indicates systolic pressure; 80 indicates diastolic pressure). Normal blood pressure changes from 20/120 in young adults to systolic pressures of 130/140 in aging patients, because of the effects of aging on the heart and arteries. Abnormally high blood pressure (e.g., 210/110) is termed *hypertension*. Abnormally low blood pressure (e.g., 80/50) is called *hypotension*. Strong emotions, pain, exercise, and some disease conditions are factors that can increase blood pressure. Resting, depression, hemorrhage, and shock are factors that can lower blood pressure. Blood pressure readings also can vary from minute to minute and day to day as a result of changes in a patient's physical, mental, or emotional activity (Rosdahl, 1985).

The volume of blood in the body and any resistance to the flow of blood through blood vessels also can affect blood pressure. For example, hemorrhaging decreases blood volume, causing the blood pressure to fall. In contrast, fatty deposits develop within the blood vessels of patients with arteriosclerosis, which causes resistance to blood flow and produces higher blood pressure readings.

The site for taking the blood pressure usually is over a large artery in the arm or leg. The brachial artery of the upper arm often is selected, but arteries of the lower arm, thigh, and calf also may be used, depending on the accessibility of the limb and the patient's condition.

When the arm is used, the patient should either sit or lie down on his/her back, with the arm and blood pressure cuff at the level of the heart.

The equipment used to measure blood pressure is a sphygmomanometer (either mercury or aneroid), a cuff, and a stethoscope (Fig. 4–2).

Mercury manometers, which provide the most accurate measurements, show increments of 10 points, from zero to 300. Aneroid manometers show units of 20, ranging from 20 to 300. The procedure is begun by raising the silver column of mercury or the aneroid needle to 200. A properly calibrated manometer will show the needle and mercury column at the zero mark on the mercury manometer (20 on the aneroid manometer) when not in use.

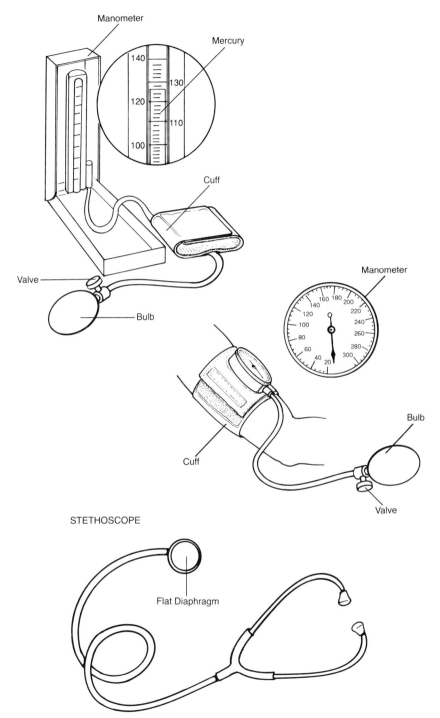

Figure 4–2. Instruments used for measuring blood pressure. Illustrates the mercury and aneroid types of manometer and the accessory equipment-(stethoscope and cuff) required to accurately measure blood pressure.

The cuff contains an inflatable rubber bladder that should be centered over the brachial artery, one inch above the elbow. Cuffs should be wrapped snugly but not tightly. If the cuff is too loose, both systolic and diastolic readings will be heard higher than their actual values (Fig. 4–3).

A stethoscope with a flat diaphragm is best for taking blood pressures. After using your fingers to locate the brachial artery in the shallow depression where the elbow bends, place the diaphragm of the stethoscope over the artery without touching the cuff or the patient's clothing. Gentle application should be used because too much pressure can cause abnormally low diastolic sounds.

Measuring blood pressure. The procedure for measuring blood pressure follows:

1. Explain the procedure to the patient in a private and noise-free environment.

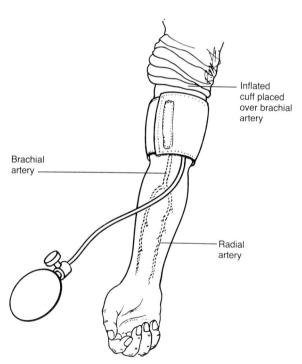

Figure 4–3. Correct positioning of the blood pressure cuff. Blood pressure cuff should be snugly wrapped approximately 1 inch above bend of arm. Stethoscope should be placed over brachial artery at bend of arm.

2. The patient should be resting for 5 minutes before the blood pressure is taken. If the patient has been actively exercising, wait 15 to 30 minutes before taking the reading.
3. Select the site and use the same site consistently because of variations in blood pressures taken in different locations. Blood pressures also should be taken with the patient in the same position each time. A lying, sitting, or standing blood pressure can vary within the same individual.
4. Remove the patient's clothing, as necessary, to expose the site. Position the patient's arm on a supporting structure (table or bed), at heart level, while the blood pressure is being taken.
5. Check to be sure that there are no leaks in the tubes, cuff, or valve.
6. Sit to take the blood pressure so that you can read the manometer at eye level. Be sure the manometer is at *zero* before beginning.
7. Let the air out of the cuff, and apply the cuff just far enough above the patient's elbow to leave the space over the brachial artery free. Wrap the cuff firmly around the patient's arm, fastening it securely on the last turn.
8. Locate the pulse in the artery, and place the stethoscope directly over the point of strongest pulsation.
9. Holding the rubber bulb in the palm of one hand, close the valve on the rubber bulb with your thumb and finger, and rapidly inflate the cuff by pumping the bulb.
10. Inflate the cuff to about 20 to 30 mm Hg above the expected systolic reading. As the cuff pressure increases, it will shut off the flow of blood within the artery. Inflation of the cuff should take 7 seconds or less.
11. Carefully loosen the valve, and deflate the cuff slowly and steadily. Listen carefully for sounds of the first heart beat (systolic pressure), and watch the mercury column or aneroid needle gauge for the points at which the sounds are first heard.
12. Deflate about 2 to 3 mm Hg per heart beat until all sounds stop or there is a distinct change in the sound (diastolic pressure). NOTE: If the cuff is deflated too slowly, false elevated readings will result. If the cuff is deflated too quickly (5 to 10 mm Hg/heart beat), false low readings will be obtained.
13. When all sounds stop, deflate the cuff rapidly and completely to zero.
14. *Do not reinflate the cuff during the reading.* If you need to repeat a reading, you must let all the air out of the cuff and wait 15 seconds before inflating the cuff again.

Interpreting arterial sounds. Arterial sounds are interpreted as follows:

1. Systolic readings are the first sound you hear as you let the air out (blood resuming flow as the heart pumps).
2. The last sound you hear as you let the air out is the diastolic reading (blood flowing freely through the artery when the heart is resting).
3. If you have difficulty hearing the diastolic sounds, completely deflate the cuff. Wait 15 seconds, and have the patient raise his or her arm to drain the blood from the blood vessels of the lower arm. When the patient lowers the arm, retake the blood pressure. NOTE: There may be distinct changes in the sounds you hear between the systolic and diastolic sounds. Sounds may become muffled before stopping or may remain muffled down to zero. In this case, record the diastolic at the point when you hear the change from clear to muffled, as well as when the sound ends completely (e.g., 120/76/62). Write down the reading promptly.
4. Repeat the procedure if you have any doubt about the reading. If the reading is elevated, wait 5 minutes and then recheck it. Briefly explain the reason for a second reading to avoid alarming the patient and affecting the blood pressure.

Patients With Tubes Or Tubing

Intravenous infusion tubing, nasogastric suction, urinary catheters, and nasal catheters and cannulas for oxygen administration are the most common types of tubing you will encounter when working with hospital patients. Although you may not be responsible for starting any of the procedures associated with such equipment, you should know how to handle and care for patients who have such tubes in place.

Intravenous equipment

Intravenous tubing, connected to a bottle or plastic bag, often is used to infuse fluids into the patient's body. A needle or plastic catheter, attached to the container, is inserted into a vein. The flow of fluid is measured by a dripmeter, and a clamp on the tubing is used to regulate the flow of the prescribed fluid (Fig. 4–4). Some institutions may use computerized infusion pumps to regulate drip rate (Rosdahl, 1985).

Unless specifically authorized, you should not change or regulate the amount of flow of a solution, even though you may have to move some patients to and from the scanning table or bed or remove their

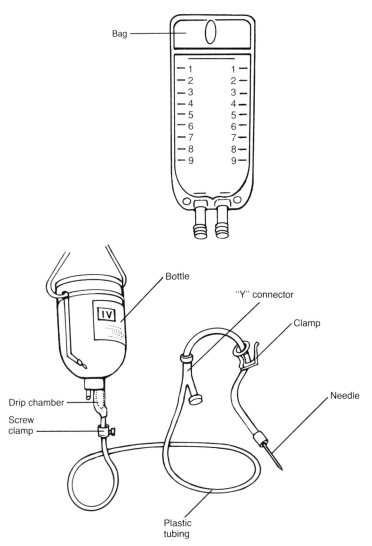

Figure 4–4. Intravenous equipment. Plastic tubing leads from a solution-filled bottle at one end and connects to a needle at the other end. Flow rate is controlled by clamping the tubing.

clothing. The following guidelines should help you in dealing with such patients.

1. If the needle has been inserted in the patient's hand or arm, help the patient keep the involved arm straight.

2. Never lower the bottle or bag below the level of the needle insertion when transferring or positioning the patient.
3. Watch for and immediately report any of the following:

- The occurrence of nausea, vomiting, rapid breathing, or an increase in pulse rate—signs of circulatory overload that must be dealt with immediately
- If no solution is passing from the bottle into the tubing even though there is still some solution in the bottle
- When the plastic drip chamber is completely filled with solution
- When you see blood in the tubing at the needle end
- When all of the solution has run out of the bottle or bag or when it is almost empty
- Whenever the needle has deliberately or accidentally been removed
- Whenever the patient complains of pain or tenderness at the needle insertion site
- Any time you notice a raised or inflamed area on the patient's skin or near the needle insertion, which may mean that the solution has *infiltrated* and is running into the adjacent tissues. (You may be requested to close the clamp to shut off the flow of solution.)
- Whenever the tubing becomes disconnected and the patient is bleeding freely from the connection site

Nasogastric tubes

It is common to see hospital patients with a tube inserted into one nostril. Depending on the length of the tube, it may terminate in the patient's stomach (i.e., a *nasogastric* tube) or intestine. Such tubes can be used for feeding, to obtain specimens, to treat intestinal obstructions, to prevent or treat distention after surgery, or to drain fluids from the patient's stomach by suction (Fig. 4–5).

When nasogastric tubing is being used to drain substances out of the stomach or to collect a specimen, the patient is given nothing by mouth (NPO) because food would only be drawn back out through the tube. In caring for patients with nasogastric tubes it is important never to pull on the tube when moving these patients or changing their positions. If the patient begins to gag or vomit while the tube is in place, *report it immediately*.

Fluids can be removed from the patient's body through the tubes by gravity or suction. The outer end of the tube may have a clamp attached, or a plastic connection may link it to longer tubing attached to an electrical suction machine. Suction (by use of either a

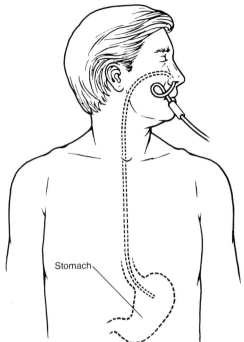

Figure 4–5. Nasogastric tube.
The nasogastric (NG) tube is inserted through one nostril and down through the esophagus until it reaches the stomach. Suction of stomach contents can be created by syringe or mechanical pump.

Stomach

syringe or a machine) often is used to remove thick secretions that cannot be drawn out easily by gravity.

Rules to follow when working with patients connected to a mechanical suction machine are as follows:

- Report any leakage in the tube or suction system.
- Never raise or open the drainage bottle.
- Never disconnect the tubing.
- Immediately report any rapid increase in the amount of material being suctioned.

Oxygen therapy

Oxygen may be administered to any patient experiencing respiratory difficulty (oxygen deficiency). The goal of such therapy is to lessen a low oxygen concentration in the blood and to decrease the workload of the respiratory system.

The use of oxygen is associated with some hazards; oxygen should be considered a drug, and its dosage or concentration should be evaluated and ordered by a physician.

Although oxygen by itself cannot burn, contact with any combustible material (even a spark) will cause it to ignite and burn or—in high concentrations—to explode.

Delivery systems for oxygen therapy include in-room piping systems and oxygen tanks, or cylinders. If your laboratory is equipped with an in-room piping system, oxygen and suction usually are provided through wall outlets. Outlet connectors, which vary in shape, color, and connection methods used, are keyed to a specific gas or function (Fig. 4–6).

Oxygen also may be contained in large tanks or in small cylinders. Large cylinders usually are used for patients requiring high flow rates or oxygen use over extended periods of time. These can be identified by size and the presence of a metal cap screwed onto the top of the cylinder to protect the valve from damage. The small cylinders are used during patient transportation or for short duration needs. The small cylinder can be identified by its size and a rectangular valve without a handle, which has three holes on one side (Rosdahl, 1985).

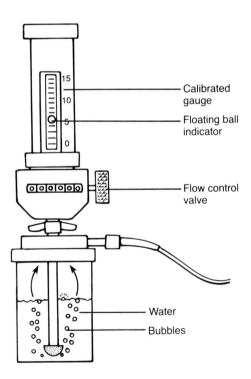

Calibrated gauge

Floating ball indicator

Flow control valve

Water

Bubbles

Figure 4–6.   Wall-mounted oxygen flowmeters. Schematic drawing of typical wall-mounted oxygen flowmeter. Water levels must be kept high enough to bubble as oxygen flows through flowmeter.

Because the gas contained within a cylinder is under extremely high pressure, the following precautions are observed whenever gas cylinders are in use:

- Never transport a high-pressure cylinder unless it is secure in a cylinder cart.
- Never allow a cylinder to stand free; it always must be secured to avoid falling and causing an accident.
- Never transport patients on a stretcher with a cylinder lying next to them.
- Never place a cylinder near a source of heat, such as a radiator, because it may cause an explosion.

The delivery of oxygen to the patient may involve the use of either high- or low-flow devices. Among the low-flow devices are the nasal cannula or nasal prongs, nasal catheter, or simple oxygen masks.

The nasal cannula is used when a patient needs extra oxygen rather than a total supply of oxygen. The prongs are inserted into the patient's nostrils and held in place by an elastic band around the patient's head. They are connected to the oxygen source by a length of plastic tubing.

A nasal catheter is a piece of tubing that is longer than a cannula. It is inserted through the nostril into the back of the patient's mouth. This method provides more effective oxygen delivery and is used when the patient must have additional oxygen at all times. The nasal catheter is fastened to the patient's forehead or cheek by a piece of adhesive tape to hold it steady.

Several different types of oxygen masks may be used. Among the most common types of masks are the following.

Simple mask. A transparent mask with a simple nipple adapter that is fitted over nose, mouth, and chin.

Partial rebreathing or reservoir mask. A low-flow device identified by the presence of a bag, which must remain constantly inflated by one third.

Venturi mask. A high-flow mask that provides the most reliable and consistent oxygen enrichment. The Venturi mask is identified by the presence of a hard plastic adapter with large "windows" on either side.

All oxygen masks, except the Venturi mask, require humidification, usually achieved by means of a humidifier (usually disposable) filled with water. The humidifier is connected to a threaded outlet at the bottom of the flowmeter or regulator. A small universal connector extends from the front or top of the humidifier for connection to the oxygen device (Rosdahl, 1985).

The following precautions should be observed in working with patients receiving oxygen therapy.

1. Observe all fire regulations in effect at your institution.
2. Check the flowmeter to be sure oxygen is being delivered to the patient. The water level in the humidifying chamber should be high enough so that it bubbles as the oxygen goes through it.
3. Be sure the tubing connected to the oxygen source is taped to the patient to help keep it from accidentally being pulled when moving the patient.
4. Make sure the patient is not lying on the tubing or that it is not kinked, which can slow or stop the oxygen flow.
5. Inhalation therapy or respiratory therapy departments are responsible in most hospitals for the patient's treatment. They should be called to make any needed adjustments after checking with the patient's physician or nurse.

Catheters

The most common kind of catheter used for removing fluids from the body is the *urinary catheter*. The catheter (made of plastic tubing) is inserted through the patient's urethra and into the bladder (Fig. 4–7). Catheters may be used to obtain sterile specimens when patients are unable to urinate naturally or to determine how much residual urine remains in a patient's bladder after urination.

A retention or indwelling catheter is a system used to provide temporary or permanent drainage of urine. A Foley catheter commonly is used. Foley catheters are specially designed as two tubes, one inside the other. The inner of the two tubes is connected at one end to a small balloon. After the catheter has been inserted, the balloon is filled with water or air so that the catheter will not pass out through the patient's urethra. Urine is drained from the bladder through the outer tube and collects in a container attached to the patient's bed or table. The flow of urine can be controlled by clamping or unclamping the tubing. It is important to note that *the catheter bag must always be positioned at a level lower than the patient's urinary bladder.* Catheterization is a sterile technique, and the catheter drainage system should consist of a closed sterile system.

As with other patient tubings, the catheter should be taped to the patient (inner thigh in this case) at all times and should be

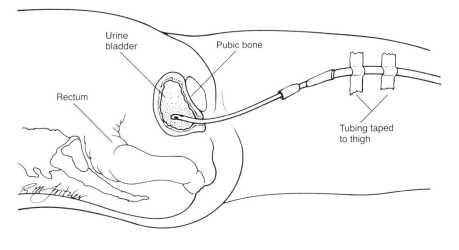

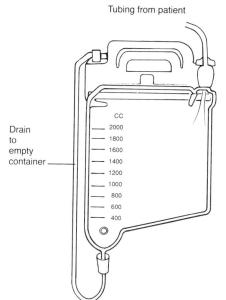

Figure 4–7. Catheterization equipment. A plastic/rubber urinary catheter is inserted through the urethra and into the bladder. Urine drains into urine container.

checked periodically for kinking or to ensure that the patient is not lying on the tubing and obstructing the flow of urine out of the body.

Another use of the urinary catheter involves patients scheduled for obstetric or gynecologic sonography. Some of these patients are unable to fill the bladder naturally and/or to maintain a full bladder for the duration of the examination. As a result they must be catheterized to instill fluid into the bladder, with the tubing clamped off until the end of the sonography study.

Because of the short length of the female urethra, the risk of urinary tract infection is increased with catheterization. For this reason it is unwise to use catheterization as a routine method of filling the bladder of patients scheduled for pelvic sonography, unless there is a *clinical* indication to do so.

Any catheterization procedure should be performed only by trained and authorized personnel.

Wound drains

After surgery a patient may have a drain or a wick placed within a wound to allow for drainage. Sonographers must anticipate and avoid the possibility of pulling or dislodging such drains during patient positioning or transfer.

Colostomies and ileostomies. Surgical treatment of patients with disorders of the intestinal tract may result in the construction of a *colostomy* (an opening into the colon) or an *ileostomy* (an opening into the ileum). In such patients, a loop of intestine is brought out of the body through a surgical incision on the abdominal wall; the opening allows drainage of feces. The colostomy or ileostomy opening (stoma) is covered by plastic disposable bags or pouches, held in place by a double-faced adhesive or special glue (Rosdahl, 1985). These appliances may require frequent changing because of the constant flow of liquid feces that is especially prevalent during the immediate postoperative period.

During abdominal sonography on such patients it is wise to have a small supply of appliances on hand because it is necessary to remove the devices to gain unobstructed access to the surface of the abdominal wall.

1. Clean rather than sterile technique is used whenever removing or changing these dressings or bags.
2. Gently remove the old appliance and cleanse the area around the stoma. Tape a folded gauze pad *around* the stoma to absorb any discharge and to protect the scanning surface during the examination.
3. Empty the contents of the old appliance into the toilet and flush. Then dispose of the old appliance in a plastic bag to prevent cross-contamination.
4. Before applying a new bag, cleanse and *dry* the skin around the

stoma so that the appliance can be securely fastened in place to prevent the escape of discharge or odors.

5. Wash your hands and clean the patient area.

Dressings. Dressings are applied as covers to wounds to protect them from further injury or infection and to absorb drainage. During the course of a sonographic examination the sonographer will be required to remove and replace dressings. Because sterile dressing changes usually are the responsibility of the nursing staff, the sonographer should always check, before removing or replacing a dressing, to determine whether wound isolation precautions are in effect. If wound isolation precautions are not required, the following steps should be carried out.

1. Wash your hands before working in the wound area. Use sterile scanning media to prevent wound infection.
2. Exercise care when removing a dressing to avoid dislodging a scab or causing the patient pain.
3. Be sure that any adhesive tape used to secure new dressings is not irritating to the patient's skin.
4. Report any unusual circumstances regarding the wound (e.g., bleeding, drainage, odor, or patient complaints of pain, burning, or itching).
5. Dispose of soiled dressings properly, and wash hands thoroughly upon completion of the patient care.

SAFETY PROVISIONS

Patient Safety

Sonographers should anticipate the safety needs of their patients, themselves, their co-workers, and their laboratory environment. You can ensure a quick response to an emergency by posting fire and disaster plans, committing them to memory, and carrying out periodic reviews.

Special precautions are needed for patients prone to medical emergencies or accidents. Knowing the location of the crash cart and other emergency equipment in your department is essential. Recognizing the fact that unconscious or sedated patients are not responsible for their own safety should prompt you to use side rails, close supervision, and restraints if necessary. Something as simple as double-checking patients' identity by matching their identification bracelets to their charts is another form of ensuring patient safety.

When performing sonography examinations on children, or when children accompany the patient to the sonography laboratory, you must consider their natural curiosity. Children's inclination to explore the environment by climbing, touching, and tasting without awareness of inherent dangers can threaten their safety.

Patients may be confused or disoriented because of medications, the effects of aging, or emotional disturbances. Such patients are not responsible for their own safety. To prepare them for any activity, always give any instructions to them clearly. Allow extra time for them to adjust to any changes in position before you require them to move.

Elderly patients may suffer from poor vision or hearing and may be unable to recognize danger or warning signals. Because their reaction times are slower than those of younger patients, they may require additional assistance in almost every physical activity.

When working with patients in wheelchairs or on stretchers, make it a practice to lock the brakes or lift the foot rests, or both. Also be sure proper body mechanics are used in transferring patients to and from wheelchairs or stretchers.

Patient safety devices frequently are used to provide postural support or restraint when patients are weakened or disabled by illness, confused by the effects of medication, or prone to accidents and injuries. If a safety device must be removed during a sonography procedure, you should ask a co-worker to help with the patient until the device is reapplied.

Treatment restraints are generally used to keep confused patients from disrupting or dislodging equipment such as intravenous or nasogastric tubes. Such restraints may take the form of mittens or soft ties around the limbs. Because the use of restraints may cause patients to feel agitated or confused by their limited ability to interact with their environment, sonographers or their delegates should stay with the patient until the person is ready to leave the sonography area.

In most institutions, restraints must be ordered by a physician or charge nurse and cannot be arbitrarily applied. Therefore it is important that both you and your patients understand that such devices are used for protection and *never as a means of punishment.*

Sonographer Safety

Often sonographers become so focused on imaging and caring for their patients that they overlook the obvious need to provide safety for themselves. Some general considerations for sonographer safety follow.

- Use good body mechanics and be sure to obtain adequate help for lifting or moving heavy objects or patients.
- Be aware of the isolation policies of your institution to protect yourself from exposure to infection.
- Ensure that electrical equipment is properly grounded for its environment.
- Avoid the use of extension cords or ungrounded adapters with electrical equipment.
- Carry out periodic inspections of cords or wires to check for fraying or defects.
- Make it a practice not to allow electrical cords to contact wet or damp areas of the patient's anatomy (e.g., gel- or oil-coated abdomen).
- Use only safety-inspected and approved devices for warming scanning media such as oils or gels; exercise extreme care if such items are "warmed" in a microwave oven.
- Remove and properly dispose of any items likely to cause accidents (e.g., needles, razor blades).
- Secure oxygen or other gas containers to prevent them from falling; prohibit smoking in areas where oxygen is used.
- Know how and where to turn in a fire alarm and where fire exits are located.

Body Mechanics

Body mechanics can be defined as the use of correct movements during the performance of any activity. Because back injuries are frequent complaints of sonographers, you need to prevent self-injury while positioning, lifting, and transporting patients in your care. Not only will good body mechanics protect you from injury, they also will reduce fatigue and allow you to use your body more efficiently and effectively. An added bonus is that the use of good body mechanics also protects your patient from injury. Initially you may find that it requires a conscious effort to maintain proper body alignment, but as you use the concept on a daily basis, it should become second nature.

Suggestions on the use of good body mechanics when lifting heavy loads follow.

1. Maintain good posture, which is essential to developing good body mechanics.

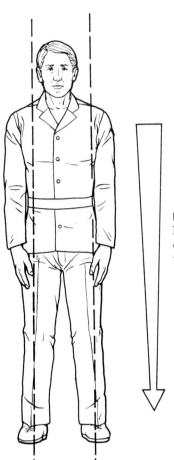

Figure 4–8. Correct posture for lifting heavy loads. Feet should be placed one shoulder length apart, with weight evenly distributed, to provide a strong support base.

2. Always evaluate a situation before acting—deciding what needs to be done and whether you will need help.
3. Always explain to patients what you plan to do.
4. Remove any objects or hazards before moving backward or during the transfer of patients.
5. Check your footing to be sure your feet are a shoulder length apart to provide a strong base of support. Distribute your weight evenly. Stand with one foot slightly forward for balance, and have the toes of the leading foot pointed in the direction of the activity (Fig. 4–8).
6. Prepare yourself for the activity by keeping your back straight and being ready to bend at the hips and knees. Use the large

muscles of the thigh instead of the smaller muscles of the back for any lifting activities. Before the lift, tighten abdominal and pelvic muscles, tuck buttocks in, and keep head and chest up.

7. Never bend sideways from the waist or hip for any activity. When turning, always pivot your feet; never twist your body.
8. Do not attempt to lift a heavy load alone if you are unsure you can do so safely.
9. Always position yourself as closely as possible to whatever you plan to lift. Never reach for a load.
10. Lift smoothly and avoid jerky movements. If lifting with the help of another person, prearrange a signal such as lifting on the count of *three*.
11. Lower your body to the object you plan to lift by bending your knees, not your back (Fig. 4–9). Straighten your legs as you lift

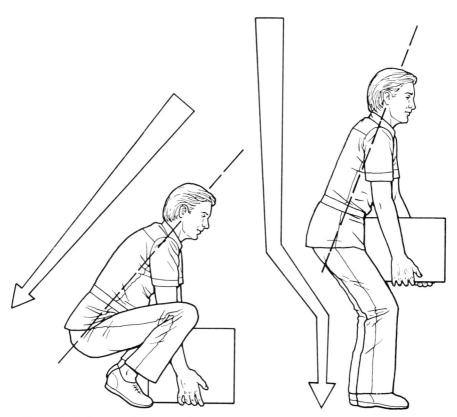

Figure 4–9. Proper body mechanics for lifting. The back should be kept straight, and the large muscles of the thigh should be used in lifting.

the object. If you must start a lift with a slightly curved back, be sure to let the large muscles of your legs take over. Whenever possible push, pull, or roll an object instead of lifting it.

Good body mechanics are equally important whenever moving, transferring, or ambulating patients. The techniques that follow can prevent injury to yourself and your patients whenever it is necessary to move them.

Moving the patient up in bed or on the scanning table

The following sequence is recommended.

1. Be sure the table or bed is locked so that it will not slide. If possible, adjust the bed to elbow height for the most comfortable position. Then relate what you are about to do, and give instructions on how the patient can help.
2. Slide or pull—rather than lift—the patient whenever possible. If the patient is unable to cooperate or is very heavy, ask a colleague to help. A lifting or turning sheet placed underneath a patient from shoulders to buttocks is helpful in such situations (Fig. 4–10).
3. Remove any pillows from the head of the table or bed, and help the patient bend the knees, with instructions to press the feet firmly on the bed.
4. Stand with one foot slightly ahead of the other as you slide one arm under the patient's shoulders and the other under the thighs. Keep the patient as close to your body as possible.
5. On the count of 3, have the patient push with the feet as you shift your weight from your back leg to your forward leg, and slide the patient up on the table or bed.
6. Replace the pillows to make the patient comfortable, and put up side rails if necessary.

Turning patients toward you

The following sequence is recommended.

1. Have the table or bed at elbow height, and stand as close to the bed as possible.
2. Using a rocking motion of your legs, shift the weight from one foot to the other as you roll the patient onto the side. Once again, a turning sheet will save time and energy.
3. When turning the patient *toward* you, check to see that the patient has ample space to turn. Then have the patient bend the knees slightly, placing the far leg over the one nearest you. Ask the

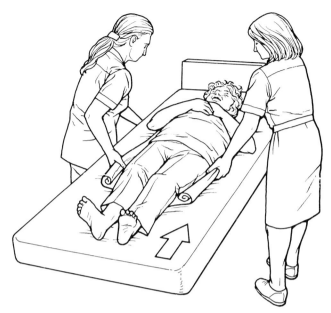

Figure 4–10. Using a lifting/turning sheet to move helpless patients. It is advisable to slide or pull, rather than to lift, helpless patients. With the help of a colleague, this technique affords the safest way to move patients who are very heavy or unable to help themselves.

patient to fold his or her hands across the chest. Place one of your hands on the patient's far shoulder and the other on the far hip, and pull the person toward you. For patients who are able to pull themselves up, you can raise the side rails for them to hold on to.

4. Maintain the patient's alignment by placing a pillow at the back to prevent the person from rolling over. Then replace the pillow under the patient's head for comfort.

Turning patients away from you

The following sequence is recommended.

1. Raise the side rails on the side the patient will turn toward.
2. Stand at the side the patient is turning from (side rails down on this side). Have the patient bend the knees slightly, placing one leg over the other so that the feet point away from you. Have the patient place folded arms across the chest.
3. Slip one of your arms under the patient's back and far shoulder. Place your other arm as far as possible under the patient's hips.

Gently roll the patient onto his or her side as you draw your arm toward you, using a rocking motion of your body and shifting your weight from your back leg to your forward leg, moving your body weight in the same direction as the patient is moving. For patients who are able to turn themselves, raise the side rails, which they can grab to pull themselves up.

4. Support the patient's alignment by placing a pillow at the back to prevent the person from rolling over. Then replace the pillow under the patient's head.

To transfer a semiambulatory or nonambulatory patient onto and off scanning tables, beds, or stretchers, as well as in and out of wheelchairs, note the following general safety considerations.

- Explain the procedure and allow the patient to help as much as possible.
- Ensure that the transfer vehicle is close to the patient and that its wheels are locked.
- Use good body mechanics, with sufficient personnel to help perform the transfer safely.
- Remember that ambulation of a person who has been in bed for prolonged periods requires a gradual approach to upright activities.

Assisting patients to and from table or bed

The following sequence is recommended.

1. Once the patient is sitting upright, move the person to the edge of the bed, with instructions to "dangle" the legs over the side of the bed (Fig. 4–11).
2. Stand facing the patient, with your weight supported evenly on both feet. Have the patient slide to the edge of the bed with the feet flat on the floor or on a stool. Give the patient a few minutes to adjust.
3. Have the patient hold onto your shoulders or—if the patient is weak—your arms. Place your hands under the patient's arms, and on the count of 3, pull the patient forward, shifting your weight from your forward foot to your backward foot (Fig. 4–12).

In assisting patients to and from a wheelchair, always keep your center of gravity at the patient's center of gravity. If patients are weak, you must control their hips and shoulders during the transfer. Do not attempt to transfer patients who are unable to bear any of their own body weight. Get help.

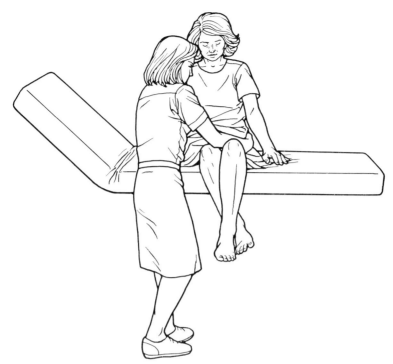

Figure 4–11. Assisting the patient out of bed or off scanning table. Always allow a weak patient to dangle the legs over the edge to regain equilibrium before attempting to move the person.

Wheelchair transfers

The following sequence is recommended.

1. Explain the procedure to the patient.
2. Position the wheelchair close to the bed, either parallel to it or at a slight angle (Fig. 4–13). Lock the wheels, and position the foot rests up and out of the way.
3. Help the patient move to the edge of the table or bed in an upright position, with legs over the edge. With the patient's hands on your shoulders, place your hands and arms under the patient's arms.
4. Assist the patient from the bed (with feet on the floor) as you rotate your weight from your forward foot to your back foot.
5. Pivot or step sideways toward the chair. Always pivot your entire body and the patient's entire body. Do not twist your back.

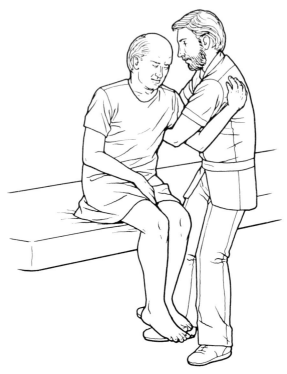

Figure 4–12. Assisting patients to and from bed or scanning table. Provide support under the arms of the patient, and rotate or shift your weight as you bring the person toward you.

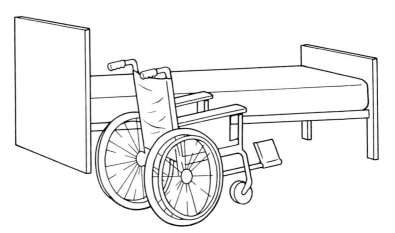

Figure 4–13. Wheelchair positioning before bedside transfer. The wheelchair should be parallel or at a slight angle to the bed, with wheels locked and footrests up and out of the way.

6. Lower the patient into the chair by lowering your body, bending at your knees and hips as the patient sits down (Fig. 4–14). Keep your shoulders level with the patient's shoulders. For patients able to help, have them grasp the arms of the wheelchair to support their own weight while sitting down and back into the chair. Once the patient is properly positioned in the chair, fold the foot rests down and position the patient's feet on the foot rests.

7. When reversing the transfer (from chair to table or bed), bring the chair next to the table/bed and lock the wheels. Lift the patient's feet, and fold the foot rests up and out of the way.

8. Have the patient place both hands on the arms of the chair; help the person stand as outlined in Figure 4–14.

9. Turn the standing patient so that his or her back is to the bed. Move the patient backward until the person is able to step up to or sit on the table/bed. Then assist the individual to lie down and swing the legs up onto the bed.

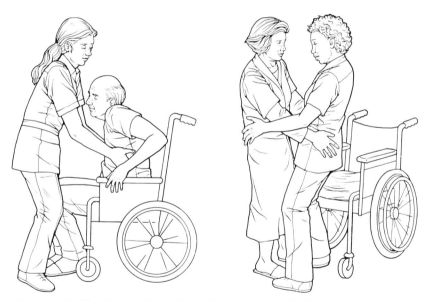

Figure 4–14. Moving patients to and from wheelchair. Bend at the knees and hips when lowering or raising a patient. Keep shoulders level with the patient's shoulders, and enlist the person's help, if possible, by having the individual support his or her own weight when rising or sitting in the wheelchair.

Stretcher transfers

The following sequence is recommended.

1. Wheel the stretcher next to the bed, aligning the head of the stretcher to the head of the bed. Move pillows and bed linens out of the way.
2. If possible, adjust the bed height to the height of the stretcher. Lock the stretcher and bed wheels.
3. Stand on the far side of the stretcher and have the patient bend the legs and place the feet flat on the bed. Instruct the patient to use the arms to help push himself or herself over and onto the stretcher.
4. For a helpless patient, position a durable sheet under the person from knees to shoulders. With the help of at least one other individual, roll the sheet close to the patient's body. Grasping the roll — on the count of 3 — lift slightly and pull the patient onto the stretcher. Be careful not to drag the patient's head (Fig. 4–15).
5. When proper positioning on the stretcher has been accomplished, cover the patient with a sheet, place a pillow under the person's head, and raise the side rails.

   NOTE: *If the patient has tubings or drains, take special care to avoid pulling them out or disconnecting them.*

Infection Control
Medical asepsis

Preventing the spread of harmful microorganisms is a basic concern in all health care settings. Microorganisms, which grow best wherever they find food, moisture, and warmth, enter the body through the nose, mouth, or breaks in the skin. Organisms also can be transported on soiled equipment and supplies, on discarded tissues and linens, and on the hands of health care professionals. For this reason, infection control is practiced in health care facilities to prevent the spread of any microorganisms considered harmful to patients and staff members. Sonographers also are expected to carry out *medical asepsis,* the technique used to prevent the spread of infections or disease.

Medical asepsis can be practiced in two ways: (1) general medical asepsis, which concerns all the measures taken to keep yourself, patients, and your environment clean to prevent the spread of germs and (2) isolation techniques and precautions that are carried out to confine disease-producing germs.

General precautions. The following precautions should be taken.

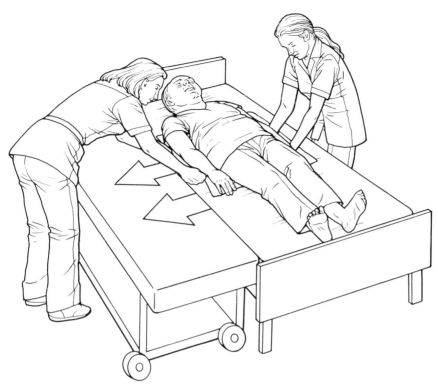

Figure 4–15. Transferring patients from bed to stretcher. Use of a "pull-ing" sheet is recommended whenever transferring patients who cannot help themselves.

- Wash your hands before and after each patient contact.
- Keep clean patient linens away from your "dirty" uniform.
- Dispose of used linens in a hamper or bag, never on furniture or the floors.
- Dispose of such items as wound dressings in the proper place.
- Keep the scanning environment clean, and allow only clean items to touch the patient.

A part of general cleanliness involves the sonographer's personal hygiene. The following checklist describes personal practices that every sonographer should observe.

- *Keep healthy.* Get adequate rest and good nutrition.
- Bathe daily and wash hair at least every week. Wear a hairstyle that is appropriate for germ control.

- Keep fingernails short, and wash hands after every patient contact.
- Wear a clean uniform or laboratory coat daily, and do not wear costume jewelry because it can harbor germs.
- Do not come to work if you are ill—especially with a communicable disease.
- Cover your mouth and nose when you cough or sneeze, and discard tissues promptly in an appropriate container.

Isolation techniques

When infections develop in patients, special steps are taken to prevent the spread of the infectious organisms. Because sonographers may be requested to perform bedside examinations of such patients or to care for patients with impaired immunity, they must understand and be prepared to follow these general isolation precautions:

1. Organize all necessary supplies before entering the patient/ isolation area to provide sonographic examinations. Working under isolation precautions can be time-consuming and frustrating; thus it is particularly important that you avoid leaving the area for forgotten supplies.
2. Wash your hands before and after each patient contact even if you wear gloves. This is the single most effective means of preventing the spread of infection. Remember, it also is important to wash your hands *again* after contact with any patient excretions or secretions before touching the patient again.
3. If you must remove dressings to perform the sonographic examination, the dressings should be properly bagged, using supplies provided within the unit.
4. All gloves used during an examination must be discarded in an appropriate container before you leave the isolation area.
5. Gowns should be discarded in a designated hamper before you leave the isolation area.
6. Masks should cover the nose and mouth and be put on before entering the isolation area, and they should be removed or discarded before leaving the isolation room. Whenever a mask becomes moist, it should be changed because it no longer provides an effective barrier to the spread of germs.
7. Masks should be used only once. Never lower your mask around your neck and then reuse it.
8. Ultrasound units must be cleansed before entering the isolation unit. Sterile transducer covers and scanning agents should be used on patients in isolation, and all equipment should be disinfected after use.

There are five specific types of isolation: strict, respiratory, enteric, wound-skin, and reverse isolation.

Strict isolation. The characteristics of this type of isolation are as follows.

- It protects others from patients' germs.
- It is used to prevent spread — by contact and/or by airborne transmission — of highly contagious diseases (such as streptococcal pneumonia, smallpox, diphtheria).
- Gowns, gloves, and masks must be worn, and all articles used must be disinfected or disposed of properly.

Respiratory isolation. The characteristics of this type of isolation are as follows.

- It protects others from germs in the patient's nose, mouth, throat, and lungs.
- It is used for diseases spread by droplets that are coughed, sneezed, or breathed into the air (such as chickenpox, mumps, tuberculosis, scarlet fever, meningococcal meningitis).
- Gowns and gloves are not necessary, but washing hands and wearing masks are required.
- Contaminated articles must be disposed of properly or disinfected.

Enteric precautions. The characteristics of these precautions are as follows.

- They protect others from germs in the patient's bowels, bladder, and stomach.
- They are used in diseases involving ingestion of disease-producing microorganisms (e.g., hepatitis, acquired immunodeficiency syndrome [AIDS]).
- Hand washing, gowns, and gloves for direct contact are necessary. Masks are not.
- Contaminated articles should be disposed of in specially provided bags, or they should be properly disinfected.

Wound-skin precautions. The characteristics of these precautions are as follows.

- They protect others from germs in patient's wounds or any other heavily contaminated areas (e.g., burns, staphylococcal or streptococcal infections).

- They are used with infections that are spread by direct contact with wounds, linens, or dressings.
- Hand washing is required, and gowns and gloves must be worn. Masks are necessary only if dressings are removed to perform the sonography examination.
- Articles contaminated with urine, feces, or vomitus should be bagged or disinfected.

Reverse (protective) isolation. Characteristics include the following.

- It protects patients from the germs of others.
- It is used with persons who have extremely impaired resistance (e.g., patients on chemotherapy, steroid therapy).
- Hand washing and the wearing of gowns, gloves, and masks are required.
- Cleansing of the ultrasound equipment and the use of sterile transducer covers and scanning media are indicated.

Emergency Medical Situations

Heart attacks and choking because of obstructed airways are frequent causes of accidental death. Choking occurs especially in children, who are known to put "everything" into their mouths. Although most sonographers perform their examinations in a medically supervised setting, it is important that they be familiar with basic lifesaving measures as they await a response to their emergency alert. If classes in lifesaving techniques are not included in your training, you may wish to investigate instructional sessions offered by the American Red Cross.

There are many reasons why a patient may experience difficulty breathing; heart attacks, strokes, seizures, and fainting are among the more common causes. You must quickly determine what has happened to your patient and then follow the general lifesaving procedures summarized here.

An agitated placement of a hand to the neck is the universal gesture of a choking person. The Heimlich maneuver (abdominal thrusts) should be performed first. If the object obstructing the person's airway is not successfully dislodged, then back slapping can be performed and the Heimlich maneuver repeated.

First aid for choking

Conscious patients. Follow these guidelines.

1. If the patient can cough, breathe, and/or talk, *do nothing.* Let the patient use his or her own coughing reflex to bring up or to clear

the airway obstruction. Otherwise you may cause the person to breathe *in* harder and force the obstructing object farther down the airway.

2. If this is unsuccessful and the patient's air is further cut off or if the person loses the ability to cough and talk, follow the procedure for the unconscious patient.

Unconscious patients. Follow these guidelines.

1. If the patient cannot talk or cough and is "wheezing" during inhalation and turning blue, perform the Heimlich maneuver. Give four quick upward thrusts to the upper portion of the abdomen (slightly above the navel). This can be done with the person standing, sitting, or lying down (Fig. 4–16).

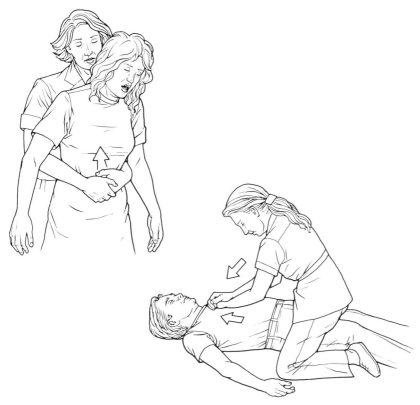

Figure 4–16. Applying the Heimlich maneuver. Abdominal thrusts may be applied to choking patients in either the standing or the supine position.

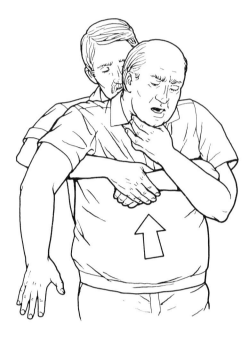

Figure 4–17. Variations on the Heimlich maneuver. Stand behind the obese or pregnant patient when performing abdominal thrusting techniques.

2. For pregnant or obese women, perform a chest thrust instead by applying pressure to the middle of the sternum and exerting a quick backward pressure to the chest (Fig. 4–17).
3. For infants and small children, turn the patient face up on your forearm with the head down. Do abdominal thrusts, using only two or three fingers (Fig. 4–18).
4. When a person begins suffering from lack of oxygen, the throat muscles relax and it may be easier to dislodge foreign objects. If the patient is unable to remove the foreign object, you can assist by grasping the patient's tongue and lower jaw with one hand and lifting up. This pulls the tongue forward and away from the back of the throat so you can see what is there. When the patient's mouth is open, insert the index finger of your other hand inside and down along the patient's cheek and deep into the throat to the base of the tongue. Using a hooking motion of the finger, dislodge the obstruction and pull it forward into the mouth where it can be removed. Be careful not to push it further down the throat.

If breathing stops and the victim appears to be unconscious, tap the victim on the shoulder and shout his or her name or *"Are you*

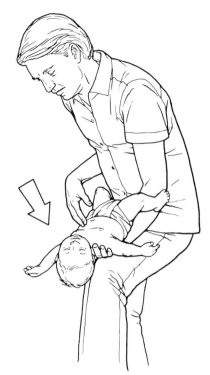

Figure 4–18. Performing the Heimlich maneuver on infants. Infants or children should be positioned face up over the forearm. Only two or three fingers should be used to perform the abdominal thrust.

okay?" If there is no response, carry out the following steps for artificial respiration.

Artificial respiration

The following procedure is recommended by the American Red Cross.

1. With the patient in the supine position, tilt the person's head, chin pointing up. Place one hand under the patient's neck and gently lift.
2. At the same time, push with the other hand on the patient's forehead. This will move the tongue away from the back of the throat to open the airway (Fig. 4–19A).
3. *Immediately look, listen, and feel for air.*
4. While maintaining the backward head tilt position, place your cheek and ear close to the patient's mouth and nose. Look for the chest to rise and fall while you listen and feel for the return of air. Check for about 5 seconds.

94

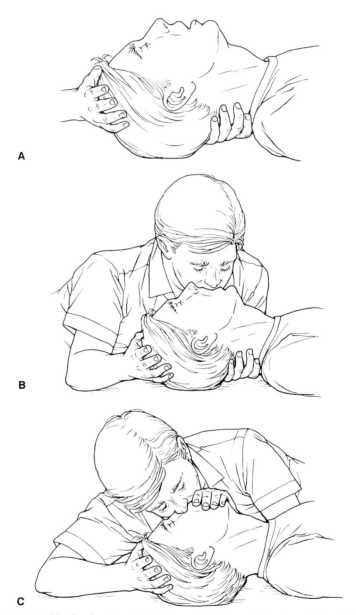

Figure 4–19. Methods of artificial ventilation. A, Backward head-tilt position. **B,** Mouth-to-mouth resuscitation technique. **C,** Mouth-to-nose resuscitation technique.

5. *If the patient is not breathing:* Maintain the backward head tilt and to prevent leakage of air, pinch the patient's nose with the hand that is on the person's forehead. Open your mouth wide, take a deep breath, seal your mouth around the patient's mouth, and blow into his or her mouth with four quick—but full—breaths, just as fast as you can. When blowing, use only enough time between breaths to lift your head slightly for better inhalation (Fig. 4–19B).

6. *For infants:* Do not tilt the head back as far as for an adult. Use gentle puffs, and blow through the mouth and nose. If you do not get an air exchange when you blow, it may help to reposition the head and try again.

7. Once again, *look, listen, and feel for air exchange.*

8. *If there is still no breathing:* Change rate to one breath every 5 seconds for an adult. For an infant, give one gentle puff every 3 seconds.

9. The *mouth-to-nose method* can be used with the aforementioned sequence instead of the mouth-to-mouth method. Maintain the backward head-tilt position with the hand on the patient's forehead. Remove the hand from under the neck and close the patient's mouth. Blow into his or her nose (Fig. 4–19C). Open the patient's mouth for the look, listen, and feel step.

Assisting Patients with Special Needs
Elderly patients

The emotional needs of the aging person are a primary concern. The emotional needs of this age-group are not really much different from those of any other, but because of the physical and social changes associated with aging, the ability to cope and maintain a positive outlook is decreased. The losses experienced by aged patients are numerous and wide-ranging: loss of spouse, family, friends, job, familiar environment, pets, and health and vigor. An accumulation of such losses can create problems in coping or adapting to change in ways that maintain independence and a sense of well-being.

The feelings of well-being, of being needed, and of loving and receiving love are diminished for the aging patient. A positive self-image, feeling important, and enjoyment of meaningful personal and interpersonal relationships are all challenged by losses.

We all accept the fact that age brings losses. Most elderly persons can cope and adapt if losses come gradually. When losses come too rapidly, however, they become overwhelming, bringing intense feelings of loneliness and frightening thoughts of loss of independence and privacy.

Sensory changes (such as diminished vision and hearing) that occur with age can lead to the inability to respond to the environment, preventing the perception of danger signals. Eventually such a lack of sensory stimulation leads to the confusion and withdrawal that is so common in elderly patients. By demonstrating concern and preparing your elderly patients for their sonograms, you will increase their feelings of control over their situation and help to decrease their level of stress.

Some memory loss is common with aging, producing slower reactions to questions, directions, and decision making. You can overcome this problem by slowing down the rate at which you give instructions, by communicating in a quiet environment with minimal activity, and by providing extra time for response.

Despite the negative aspects of aging, there are many potential rewards in dealing with elderly patients. A lifetime of living has given them a wealth of knowledge and experience; thus asking their opinions or advice can result in useful suggestions concerning what will work best for them. Elderly patients provide sonographers a chance to practice the almost lost art of listening, if we just encourage them to talk about their experiences. Talking about their experiences and accomplishments makes them feel that their lives had a purpose. By boosting their self-esteem and independence, you can make the elderly patient a more cooperative patient.

Touching, and receiving affection, are very important. A smile, a pat on the arm, or a squeeze of the hand are just as essential as food and shelter; these gestures help to ease the loss of human contact that relocation or death may have brought into the lives of elderly patients.

Patience, caring, and sensitivity are the keys to working with all patients, but especially with the elderly. It is important to respect and treat them as adults—not children. By planning your examination with their individual needs in mind, everyone will benefit from the experience.

Transcultural Backgrounds

Only recently has the medical community begun to realize the full impact of a patient's culture on recovery. In some cultures illness is looked upon as the will of God or as a punishment for sins. In others, illness is attributed to outside forces.

Ethnicity. Beliefs about nutrition and dietary practices and about illness and its causes and cures, as well as religious beliefs aboutillness and death, are just as important as special anatomic considerations or disorders specific to a particular cultural group.

In working with patients from other cultures and backgrounds, it is easy to develop cultural biases because of language barriers, physical appearances, or differing religious beliefs and mores. A *cultural bias* is a tendency to interpret words or actions according to some culturally derived meaning assigned to it (Purtilo, 1984). Identifying a cultural bias was once easy because our patient populations were relatively homogeneous and we were comfortable doing things the *American* way. Today, however, with the arrival of increasing numbers of emigrants and refugees, America has become multicultural — more a part of the global village of our planet. Consequently, sonographers must develop an understanding of transcultural variables and their effects (Rosdahl, 1985) (Table 4–2).

Treatments and cures vary widely from one cultural group to another. Black and Latino cultures have long used roots, potions, and herbs for treating sickness. Some credit the use of charms, amulets, and faith healers with driving away evil spirits. Native American women do not seek early prenatal care because they believe that pregnancy is a natural, normal process. To many transcultural patients, a hospital or clinic is associated with illness and death. Once you recognize the roles that cultural differences can play, you will begin to understand why your former patients may have reacted inappropriately to your concept of "normal."

Religion. Religious beliefs about illness can play strong roles in the reactions of Jews, Roman Catholics, Mormons, Christian Scientists, Seventh-Day Adventists, and Jehovah's Witnesses. Such religions may dictate behaviors of wide-ranging impact on the patient's diet, consideration of abortion, or acceptance of medication, treatments, or surgery.

Distance and time. One evident area of cultural bias concerns the distance people believe is appropriate when communicating and physically interacting with one another. Americans generally divide distance into four zones: intimate, personal, social, and public (Hall, 1966). Such biases are significant to sonographers because sonography procedures take place within such personal and intimate zones. Imagine how a patient from another culture might resent being "embraced" by a sonographer who was merely trying to assist them onto the scanning table. In contrast, there also are cultures in which patients refuse even to speak to a sonographer unless they are literally toe-to-toe and would be offended by a sonographer who unwittingly stepped back or withdrew from them. Patients who regard distances differently than we do expect us to respect their customs.

Time. The *right time* and the *correct time* are not always synony-

Table 4–2. Transcultural Patient Variables

Variable	Explanation
Cultural background	Differences and similarities between patient and sonographer
Definitions	Specific cultural definitions and concepts relating to health and the causes of illness and injury
Medical practices	"Folk medicine" or tribal practices
Attitudes	Customs and practices regarding health care, relationships, and interactions (e.g., personal space, eye contact, modesty)
Socioeconomic status	Economic level of patients or family
Environmental factors	Contributing factors, such as substandard nutrition and housing, that may affect the patient's chief complaint or related disorders
Terminology	Specific names, terms, or slang related to illness (e.g., "bad blood," "proud flesh," "mal ojo")
Language barriers	Differences in language of patient/family and sonography staff
Body concepts	Attitudes regarding nudity/modesty; male-female interactions
Physical/health concepts	Reactions to pain, aging, death, childbirth, abortion, mental retardation, or mental illness
Moral-ethical concepts	Attitudes regarding sexual expression, homosexuality, incest, or illegitimacy
Dietary customs	Religious or cultural concepts about food and how they relate to specific illnesses; dietary taboos
Physical appearance	Attitudes about obesity; adaptability to special therapeutic diets; cleanliness and grooming
Religion	Importance of religious beliefs and practices

Modified from Rosdahl, C. B.: Textbook of Basic Nursing, 4th ed. New York: J. B. Lippincott Co., 1985.

Table 4–2. **Transcultural Patient Variables** *Continued*

Variable	Explanation
Group identity	Importance and type of family structure; traditional male-female roles
Visible differences	Physical differences related to ethnic background (e.g., black, Native American, Oriental)
Inherited conditions	Disorders specific to cultural groups (e.g., sickle cell anemia, Tay-Sachs disease)
Demographics	Number of people belonging to a group in the same geographic area as the health care facility
Prejudices	Within the same cultural group or directed to "outsiders"; stereotyping of other cultural-ethnic groups
Racial-cultural differences	Mixed families: mixed races, religions, or cultural backgrounds

mous to all patients. Although most American sonographers are compulsively punctual and expect their patients to be the same, in some South American and South African cultures an appropriate amount of tardiness is considered normal. The result is that such patients feel no obligation to apologize for being late. In fact they would be offended if a sonographer appeared rushed or hurried during their examination and would consider such behavior insulting.

The American concept of "first come, first served" also is alien to cultures in which the oldest or the sickest patients are seen first or in which the highest-ranking patients or female patients receive preferential treatment.

Cultural biases can be so deep-seated that individuals are not consciously aware that they have them; thus it will take an astute sonographer to recognize and consider such facts when attempting positive patient interactions.

Religious and ethnic mores may play an important role whenever sonographers are asked to perform highly intimate examinations involving the heart or reproductive organs. Male sonographers in particular face such biases more frequently than do their female counterparts. If the patient's reluctance to submit to such sonographic examinations cannot be overcome, it may be necessary for the sonographer to call in a chaperone or to trade places with a physician or another sonographer of an acceptable gender.

Prejudice. Another form of culturally derived bias is prejudice. It may be based on race, ethnicity, or appearance. As a sonographer, you must be constantly aware of the injurious effects of such discrimination and thus make every effort to understand the personal biases of your patients, as well as your own. In some cases, you may even be expected to defuse potentially hostile situations for those who cannot overcome such feelings.

PART II
Basic Sonographic Techniques

LEARNING OBJECTIVES
Students who successfully complete this unit will be able to:

- List the major specialty sonographic examinations.

- Describe/demonstrate the standard patient positions relative to sonographic imaging.

- Discuss patient preparations for abdominal, obstetric-gynecologic, and cardiac sonography.

- Describe the basic components of the three major specialty scanning protocols.

It is common medical practice to organize patients into groups such as medical-surgical, obstetric, pediatric, geriatric, or psychiatric. In sonography it also is common to categorize sonographic examinations by the clinical area or specialty to which they correspond.

Initially, sonographers were expected to perform all of the existing forms of specialty examinations. As the field expanded and sophisticated equipment and techniques were developed, however, this "jack of all trades" concept changed. Today most sonographers choose to specialize in one or more of the following clinically identified examinations:

- Neurosonography
- Ophthalmologic sonography
- Vascular sonography
- Cardiac sonography (adult and pediatric)
- Abdominal sonography
- Obstetric sonography
- Gynecologic sonography
- High-resolution sonography (superficial structures, intraoperative techniques)

This portion of Unit Four focuses on the three most widely practiced diagnostic ultrasound specialties: abdominal sonography, obstetric and gynecologic sonography, and cardiac sonography.

SCANNING TECHNIQUE

The major goal of sonographers is to master proper sonographic techniques to ensure the production of high-quality diagnostic sonograms and minimal patient discomfort. To acquire proficiency in performing sonographic examinations, it is understood that a sonographer must possess an adequate knowledge of anatomy, disease processes, and sonographic data (Table 4–3). The evolution of today's high-resolution real-time equipment, however, requires sonographers to bring much more than a systematic approach to scanning if they are to avoid missing or overlooking adjacent or associated pathologic conditions. It no longer is sufficient simply to manipulate transducers, make measurements, and record images. Competent sonographers also are expected to have an excellent understanding of the common diseases and to recognize any situation that calls for unusual views or patient preparations. In addition, they are required to use skill in compiling clinically relevant data through chart reviews, obtaining additional history and physical data if necessary, and communicating (in verbal or written form) their observations of the manner in which ultrasound energy penetrated and reflected back from the patient's tissues.

As you progress through your training, you will receive in-depth instructions on how to perform correct sonographic examinations of the many organs and systems of the body. What follows here should be considered a simple introduction to those complex activities, which, along with continuing study and personal experience, will expand your potential and value as a respected member of the diagnostic team. *Text continued on p. 106*

Table 4–3. Sonographic Strategies in Relation to Common Chronic Illnesses

ARTHRITIS

Definition

Inflammatory disease of the joints

Symptoms

Joint pain or stiffness (especially in the morning); as disease progresses, joint deformities increase while movement may be severely limited and painful.

Scanning strategies

- Warmth is soothing. Be sure patient has adequate coverings.

- Avoid applying excess transducer pressure in area of painful joints.

- Include time for rest periods during the sonographic examination so that patient may exercise immobilized joints.

CANCER

Definition

Growth of abnormal cells to form masses that may alter normal body functions and can lead to death

Symptoms

Depend on location of tumor. General symptoms are unexplained weight loss; unusual bleeding; palpable lump; sore that will not heal; difficulty in swallowing; change in bowel/bladder habits; change in appearance of warts or moles.

Scanning strategies

- Encourage patient to get/continue medical care early.

- Use a stand-off scanning device if patient has fresh surgical incisions.

- Offer emotional support and encourage patient to express feelings.

DIABETES

Definition

Pancreatic dysfunction that results in inadequate insulin production; linked to serious congenital abnormalities in the pregnant patient

Symptoms

Thirst, weight loss; headaches; constant hunger and fatigue; poor circulation; hardening of the arteries; prone to infections

Table 4–3. Sonographic Strategies in Relation to Common Chronic Illnesses *Continued*

Scanning strategies

- In pregnant diabetic patients, perform meticulous scans of the fetus to detect possible cardiovascular, gastrointestinal, or genitourinary skeletal abnormalities.

- Encourage patients to continue medications or other therapies.

EMPHYSEMA

Definition

Loss of alveolar elasticity resulting in breathing difficulties

Symptoms

Shortness of breath and difficulty breathing; patient may require upright or "bent over" position to facilitate breathing.

Scanning strategies

- Accommodate patient positional needs at all times during sonography examination.

- Encourage patient to breathe out through pursed lips to exhale all air between inspirations.

- Administer oxygen only under supervision of physician or nurse.

- Allow patient to rest during examination.

MULTIPLE SCLEROSIS

Definition

Disease of the nervous system causing gradual degeneration

Symptoms

Paralysis/numbness of extremities. Blindness, deafness, and speech and mental problems may occur. Severe disease progresses to permanent disability.

Scanning strategies

- Ensure safety of patient (such as side rails up).

- Evaluate what abilities the patient has retained.

- Arrange for bladder filling by catheterization for gynecologic studies.

- Assist ambulatory patients *at all times*.

Table continued on following page

Table 4–3. Sonographic Strategies in Relation to Common Chronic Illnesses *Continued*

ORGANIC BRAIN DISEASE

Causes

Lack of oxygen to the brain, alcoholism, Alzheimer's disease, senile dementia

Symptoms

May be mild, moderate, or severe, including impaired orientation, memory, or judgment. Difficulty in learning new things or taking direction. Shows little emotion to frequent changes of emotion. With severely impaired brain function, the patient may lose contact with reality and suffer hallucinations or react inappropriately.

Scanning strategies

- Provide for patient safety if patient is confused or forgetful.

- Be patient and understanding. Be willing to repeat instructions.

- Try to provide social, emotional, and reality stimulation while the patient is in your care.

PARKINSON'S DISEASE

Definition

Disease of the basal ganglia that governs movement; usually occurs in later years of life

Symptoms

Shuffling gait, finger tremors, muscular weakness, rigid, bent posture; no alteration in mental or intellectual functioning

Scanning strategies

- Provide for patient safety. Keep traffic areas free of clutter to prevent falls. Assist patient onto scanning table.

- Encourage patient activity during scanning "rest periods" to maintain mobility.

- Provide emotional support.

SPINAL CORD INJURIES

Definition

Traumatic injury to the spinal cord resulting in varying degrees of paralysis; paralysis of the legs (paraplegia) or of the arms and legs (quadriplegia)

Table 4–3. Sonographic Strategies in Relation to Common Chronic Illnesses *Continued*

Symptoms

Paralysis occurs below the level of the injury. Patient may have respiratory problems because of diaphragmatic paralysis or bowel/bladder incontinence in association with lower level paralysis.

Scanning strategies

- Patient will require transfer and/or ambulation assistance. Anticipate the need to have a co-worker available to help with these activities.

- May suffer from ileus and require enemas as an abdominal sonography preparation.

STROKE

Definition

A cerebral vascular accident (CVA) resulting from blockage or rupture of the blood supply to specific areas of the brain

Symptoms

Variable, ranging from minor to severe depending on severity of blood flow interruption: confusion, slurred speech, headaches, vision problems, weakness of an arm or a leg. Patients may lose sensation on the affected side; may have difficulty swallowing and/or eating. Stroke victims frequently experience memory loss of recent events and have difficulty remembering directions. Such complications or immobility from contractures or pressures sores can develop if the patient does not receive proper care.

Scanning strategies

- Provide emotional support to patients with speech/vision problems, inasmuch as they easily become frustrated.

- Take safety precautions to prevent falls.

- Anticipate the need to have a co-worker available to help move the patient.

- Approach patients with vision problems *head on,* and announce who you are.

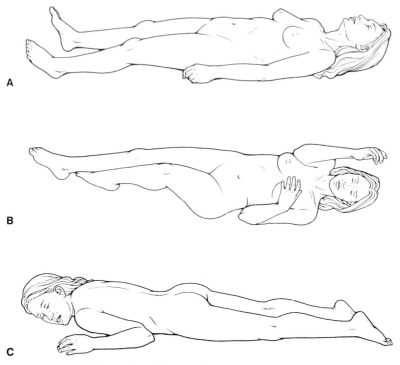

Figure 4–20. Primary imaging positions. A, Supine; **B,** lateral; **C,** prone.

SONOGRAPHIC POSITIONING

An important part of performing sonography examinations involves correctly positioning the patient and knowing when a position change can enhance the visualization of an area of interest. Figure 4–20 depicts the patient positions most commonly used in sonography.

Supine

This position also is referred to as the dorsal recumbent position. The patient lies on his or her back with head and upper shoulders slightly elevated to provide comfort and to maintain the natural curve of the spine at the neck. A small pillow placed under the knees will relieve pressure on the patient's back. The patient's arms should be positioned at the side or across the chest.

For examinations of the upper portion of the abdomen, the patient's right arm is elevated to expand the rib spaces to their fullest. This permits placement of small, narrow-faced transducers within the intercostal spaces and improves both transmission and reflection of the sound beam by eliminating rib artifacts.

Lateral

The patient lies on his or her side with arms positioned in front. The dependent arm may be elevated toward the head, and the other arm is crossed over the chest. The dependent leg should be straight, and the other leg should cross over so that the knee comes to rest on the table top, supporting the patient.

Prone

The patient lies on his or her abdomen, arms flexed at either side or elevated alongside the head to widen the intercostal spaces. A small pad or pillow placed under the patient's head, abdomen, and lower legs will relieve pressure. The patient's feet should extend off the scanning table.

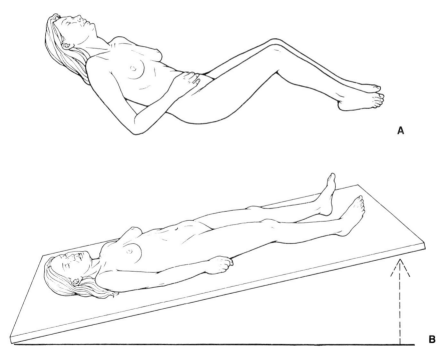

Figure 4–21. Secondary imaging positions. A, Modified Fowler: Head elevated approximately 25 degrees. Knees slightly flexed. **B,** Trendelenburg: Patient's pelvis positioned higher than her head.

Variations

Several position variations may be indicated during the course of an examination. These include the upright, modified Fowler's, and Trendelenburg's positions (Fig. 4–21).

Upright position. The patient sits on the edge of the scanning table, right arm elevated above the head, left arm and hand providing support. This position is helpful in scanning a gallbladder in an extremely high position under the rib cage.

Modified Fowler. This position is useful in advanced pregnancy when elevation of the patient's head and upper portion of the back is necessary to avoid vena caval hypotension.

Trendelenburg. The patient's pelvis is elevated 20 to 30 per cent by means of tilting the lower portion of a scanning table or the use of pillows or foam bolsters. This position is used whenever fetal parts obscure the lower uterine segment or the fetal lie prevents suitable imaging of the fetal head.

PATIENT PREPARATION FOR SONOGRAPHY EXAMINATION

The general considerations when preparing a patient for sonography examination are as follows:

- To inform patient of the purpose of the test
- To prepare the patient (e.g., disrobing, positioning, applying scanning media)
- To obtain patient history (also brief physical examination if indicated)
- To review sonographic techniques pertinent to the clinical request.

MAJOR SONOGRAPHIC EXAMINATIONS

Abdominal Sonography

The following outline presents the accepted procedure in abdominal sonography.

I. Preliminary steps
  A. Explain the purpose of the examination to the patient.
  B. Confirm that the patient's preparation (fasting or hydrating stomach or bladder) has been carried out.
  C. Obtain patient history pertinent to the organ/system to be evaluated.

    1. Query the existence of the following symptoms or complaints: right or left upper quadrant pain, fullness, fever, abdominal pain, nausea, or vomiting
    2. Symptoms related to certain types of food (e.g., fatty foods, fried foods); presence of midabdominal pain, burning, belching, or regurgitation
    3. Flank pain, urinary tract symptoms (e.g., hematuria, bacteremia)

II. Medical history
    A. Infectious diseases (such as mononucleosis, hepatitis)
    B. Alcohol intake
    C. History of carcinoma (personal)
    D. Family history of carcinoma, alcoholism, blood disorders (e.g., leukemia, anemia, tuberculosis, syphilis)

III. Present medications
    A. Ulcer medication or antacids
    B. Antidepressants
    C. Antiarrhythmic agents
    D. Cholesterol-lowering agents

IV. Laboratory data: awareness of normal values and the function of the following tests
    A. Serum glutamic-oxaloacetic transaminase (SGOT) (aspartate aminotransferase, AST)
    B. Serum glutamate pyruvate transaminase (SGPT) (alanine aminotransferase, ALT)
    C. Alkaline phosphate
    D. Bilirubin
    E. Blood-urea-nitrogen (BUN)
    F. Urinalysis

V. Review of basic scanning protocols
    A. Patient positions: supine, left/right lateral (decubitus), prone, or erect
    B. Transducer selection (based on patient's body habitus and examination objectives)
    C. Acoustic scanning media (gel, water, oil)
    D. Imaging modalities (e.g., film, tape)
    E. Scanning planes: longitudinal, transverse, coronal, and oblique

Obstetric-Gynecologic Sonography

The following outline presents the accepted procedure in obstetric-gynecologic sonography.

I. Preliminary steps
   A. Explain purpose of procedure to patient.
   B. Check that patient preparation (full bladder/empty bladder) has been carried out.
II. Patient history
   A. Establish parity and date of last menstrual period (LMP) and/or estimated date of confinement (EDC).
   B. Past reproductive history.
   C. General physical status, and past or current history:
      1. Hypertension
      2. Sequelae
      3. Diabetes
      4. Rh isoimmunization
      5. Thyroid abnormality
      6. Heart disorders
      7. Hepatitis
      8. Herpes type II
      9. AIDS
      10. Cigarette smoking
      11. Alcohol
      12. Medications
      13. History of thrombophlebitis
      14. History of miscarriage, abortion, infertility, multiple births, prior surgery, or congenital anomalies
III. Laboratory data, including tests such as the following:
   A. Human chorionic gonadotropin (HCG) (quantitative HCG assay)
   B. Amniotic fluid analysis
   C. Chorionic villus sampling (CVS)
   D. Alpha-fetoprotein (AFP) assay
   E. Percutaneous umbilical blood sampling (PUBS)
   F. Estrogen and progesterone levels
IV. Review of basic scanning protocols
   A. Transducer selection based on patient contours and desired field of view
   B. Selection of scanning agent
   C. Selection of imaging/recording modality
   D. Patient positions: longitudinal; transverse coronal and oblique

Cardiac Sonography

The following outline presents the accepted procedure in cardiac sonography.

I. Preliminary steps
   A. Inform patient of purpose of the test.
   B. Instruct patient to disrobe from chest to waist.
II. Patient history
   A. Chief complaint and location of complaint
   B. Present illness: onset, duration, precipitating condition(s)
   C. Current medications: antihypertensives, antiarrhythmics, anticoagulants
   D. Known allergy to medications: digitalis, nitrates, beta blockers, diuretics
   E. Cardiac symptoms: chest pain, dyspnea, orthopnea, fatigue, cough, edema, syncope, dizziness, palpitations, fever, cyanosis, ascites
   F. Previous conditions: hypertension, myocardial infarction, rheumatic fever, diabetes, heart murmur, endocarditis, pericarditis, cardiomyopathy, pulmonary disease
   G. Previous cardiac surgery: coronary artery bypass graft, valve replacement (mitral, aortic, tricuspid, or pulmonic)
   H. Social history: use of cigarettes, alcohol, drugs (e.g., cocaine, other narcotics)
III. Physical examination
   A. Obtain blood pressure readings in both arms while patient is in the supine, sitting, and standing positions.
   B. Auscultate lung fields (optional).
   C. Perform cardiac auscultation
      1. Determine heart sounds: systolic and early/late diastolic filling sounds; low-pitched sounds; midsystolic clicks; pericardial rubs; coarse systolic murmurs; high-pitched, blowing murmurs.
      2. Determine other diastolic sounds and murmurs.
IV. Review of basic scanning protocols
   A. Positioning: supine, lateral, erect
   B. Transducer selection based on patient's body habitus and examination objectives
   C. Acoustic scanning media
   D. Scanning planes: intercostal, subcostal, suprasternal

SUMMARY

After completing this unit, it should be apparent that the role of a sonographer is much more complex than simply functioning as a picture-taker and minor functionary on the diagnostic team. Sonographers must also deliver appropriate basic care to the patients entrusted to them. The patient should emerge as the pivotal point of interest, deserving of the best the medical profession has to offer.

As members of the diagnostic team, sonographers expect to work toward mastering the technical skills that are demanded of them. However, they should never lose sight of the fact that maintaining or restoring the patient to health is their ultimate goal.

This knowledge should prompt sonographers to show consideration for patients' emotional and physical condition, to accept the responsibility of learning basic patient care, and to demonstrate an unconditional acceptance of and respect for the ethnic and cultural differences between their patients and themselves.

REFERENCES

Burke, S. B.: Human Anatomy and Physiology for the Health Sciences, 2nd ed. New York: John Wiley & Sons, 1980.

Hall, E. T.: The Hidden Dimension. New York: Doubleday & Co., 1966.

Purtilo, R.: Health Professional/Patient Interaction, 3rd ed. Philadelphia: W. B. Saunders Co., 1984.

Rosdahl, C. B.: Textbook of Basic Nursing, 4th ed. New York: J. B. Lippincott Co., 1985.

▼

U N I T   5

Communication Skills and Problem Solving

LEARNING OBJECTIVES

Students who successfully complete this unit will be able to:

• Define communication and the components necessary for communication to occur.

• Compare and contrast verbal and nonverbal communication

• Identify at least three barriers to communication.

• Differentiate supportive from social forms of conversation.

• Describe the type of responses that are most likely to cut off communication.

• Discuss various approaches used in communicating with patients who require special assistance.

• List the advantages and disadvantages of sonographer reports, including the creation of images (films and tapes) for patient use.

Communication can be defined as the exchange of information, which is accomplished by sending and receiving messages. True communication, however, is more. It includes the ability to receive, interpret, and respond appropriately and clearly to messages. To be effective communicators, sonographers must develop not only communication skills but the ability to listen and convey interest, compassion, knowledge, and information.

COMMUNICATION CHARACTERISTICS

Several components are required for communication to occur:

- A sender (the originator of the message or idea)
- A message channel (verbal or nonverbal means of transmitting the message or idea)
- A receiver (someone to receive and interpret the message)
- An interaction (feedback that results from the receiver's response)

Communication is successful only when both the sender and the receiver understand the message the same way. In effective communication, senders and receivers often use both verbal and nonverbal communication. *Verbal* communication includes the transmission of words in either verbal or written form, whereas *nonverbal* communication consists of eye contact, facial expressions, body movements and posture, tone of voice, and touch. In some instances, the message the patient wishes to impart is contradicted by the accompanying nonverbal "expressions." As a worker in the health care profession, you will find yourself involved in many types of communication.

Social conversation is an automatic type of communication that we use out of habit. Usually consisting of polite or friendly exchanges of factual or social information, such conversation is superficial and flows easily from one topic to another. Social conversation does not provide significant information, identify problems, nor result in solutions. Nevertheless, social conversation is important in establishing a relationship with patients and creating a climate for more supportive communication.

Supportive conversation is more goal-oriented than is social conversation. Important patient information is discussed — how patients feel and any problems that concern them can be shared. The purpose of supportive conversation is to help relieve patient anxiety, anger, or frustration and to learn about any unmet patient needs. By talking through such concerns, it often is possible to help patients resolve their problems. However, supportive conversation can be successful only if the sonographer really understands the patient and facilitates that understanding by means of the following skills:

- *Listening* carefully to the message as well as the words that the patient is speaking.
- *Observing* any nonverbal communications that the patient may be sending. Sometimes this type of communication is more accurate than the verbal message. For example, when patients are eager to

communicate, they maintain eye contact. Lack of eye contact often represents uncomfortable emotions such as anxiety, depression, and embarrassment. Body language in the form of yawning, drumming the fingers, shrugging the shoulders, or rolling the eyes sends the message "I'm uncomfortable," "I'd rather not be here," or "Hurry up!" Sonographers must be sensitive to the feelings that patients express by both words and actions.

- *Responding appropriately.* Patients feel more at ease in talking about their problems and concerns when the listener exhibits attentiveness and interest. Anything you say to the patient should relate to what the patient has just told you, either verbally or nonverbally. Providing feedback encourages patients to keep talking about their concerns until they have talked them out or reached some decisions.
- *Maintaining silence.* Allow patients and yourself to be silent in order to give the patient the chance to decide what to say or not to say. Evaluate the silence. Is it heavy, sad, tense, or comfortable? Silence also can mean that the patient does not want to talk anymore. We must impress upon our patients that that is okay, too.
- *Clarifying.* Check the statements you heard or the cues you observed to be sure you know what they mean. It is very important that patients know you understand their communications. It also is important to avoid ambiguity because it creates communication problems.
- *Repeating.* Repeating ideas or statements the patient has communicated clarifies the message and also allows patients to change their mind or to reinforce their viewpoints.
- *Gathering information.* Attempt to obtain as much information about patients as possible by asking questions that are open-ended and cannot be answered with a simple yes or no response.
- *Summarizing.* By verbally listing or reviewing the ideas that patients express, you allow them to take a more objective look at their comments. This can be especially helpful with patients who have difficulty making decisions.
- *Accepting.* Patients should be encouraged to express negative feelings or thoughts even if you disagree. It is important not to be judgmental or to convey that impression through words, facial expressions, or body language.
- *Touching.* A pat on the shoulder or a touch on the hand are nonverbal gestures of support. Just be sure that your patient does not have any objections to being touched.

FACTORS IN COMMUNICATION

Barriers

Anything that interferes with the communication process constitutes a barrier. Both verbal and nonverbal barriers exist, and they can be communicated either by senders or by receivers. One common barrier is talking too fast. Using slang, medical vocabulary, or broad generalizations also can make it difficult for the receiver to know what the sender is trying to say.

Sonographers must avoid "talking down" to patients or speaking in hostile or insulting tones. Such behavior makes patients defensive and unable to understand messages. Strong feelings such as anger or prejudice toward the person who is speaking also can cause misunderstanding of what is being said. Listeners often miss parts, or all, of a message when they are distracted by their concern about their problems. Labeling patients as "complainers" or "disoriented" will only encourage listeners to ignore or misunderstand what that patient is saying (Craig, 1987a; 1989).

Language can be a communication barrier if the sender and receiver speak different languages. Keep in mind that smiling is a universal language technique, and use hand signals if possible. If you try to speak a few words in the other person's language, it will be appreciated and will gain you cooperation.

Cutting Off Communication

Whenever a listener prevents a conversation from starting or continuing, or moving from a social to a supportive level, the communication is cut off. Common reasons why listeners do this are embarrassment, feeling threatened, or distrust of the sender. Such tactics may be either conscious or subconscious.

The following examples are responses that will stop or cut off communication.

- *Judgmental responses.* Telling patients they should not feel angry or afraid or that you know of people in worse situations can only leave the patient feeling guilty or ashamed for complaining.
- *Arguing.* Debating with patients instead of learning what they are thinking is counterproductive.
- *Solving.* Avoid offering advice or answers before patients have the chance to think of their own solutions.
- *Interrupting.* Cutting off patients before they have a chance to have their say puts you at risk for receiving only part of the message and giving an inappropriate response.

- *Changing the subject.* Patients feel that you do not want to listen to them when you deliberately change the subject before a topic is completed.
- *Distractions.* Sonographers must guard against showing (by body language or behavior) that they are disinterested.
- *False assurances.* Kidding or falsely cheering patients out of a situation makes only you feel more comfortable. It deprives the patient of working through a problem and possibly finding solutions or making decisions.
- *Untruthfulness.* Never fabricate or construct excuses to avoid confronting patients with unpleasant news.
- *Evasion.* Do not focus patients' attention on their signs or symptoms simply to reassure them or to avoid being questioned about whether they are going to die.
- *Avoidance.* Do not redirect patient questions to someone else, thereby indicating that you cannot or will not answer.
- *False reassurance.* Avoid telling patients not to worry—that everything will be all right—just to prevent them from talking about their fears. You really do not know that everything will be fine. By saying these things, you may prevent patients from working through their fears or working out solutions to their problems. Instead show respect for patients by a willingness to listen without judgment to their concerns and feelings. Give correct information that is as true and as factual as possible. If you do not know the facts, or are not free to discuss them, find someone who is authorized to give that information. Your patients must trust your honesty (Craig, 1989).

Exploring Attitudes and Feelings

A patient's physical state (such as being tired, cold, rested) or emotional state (such as being sad, happy, confident) can greatly affect the ability to carry on a supportive conversation. Both sonographers and patients can be affected. A sonographer who does not feel well may become irritated by the patient's behavior and not really listen to—may even avoid—the patient. When patients do not feel well, they often become angry or stubborn. It is helpful in such instances to realize that this may not be the right time to work out a problem. If you become aware that this is happening, take a break, seek help, and try to be careful about what is said. Strong negative emotions such as anger and crying are particularly difficult to handle in such circumstances.

Realize that these same situations can occur between you and your co-workers, your family, or friends. When problems cannot be resolved, when you sense hard feelings or anger among your co-workers, when you cannot seem to communicate with your supervisor—step back and evaluate the situation. Take a look at what happens when you talk to each other and how each of you feels about yourself and the other person. You can use the same techniques of developing a supportive conversation to help you communicate effectively with co-workers, family, and friends, as well as with patients.

PATIENTS WITH SPECIAL COMMUNICATION PROBLEMS

The ability to communicate relies heavily on our five senses, especially hearing, seeing, and touching. Patients who cannot hear or see not only have difficulty communicating but also may become confused. When dealing with patients with any sensory losses, sonographers should plan to use the patient's remaining senses to their fullest.

In working with elderly or hospitalized patients, you may encounter confusion. The causes of the patient's confusion may range from too little stimulation of the patient's five senses to physical causes such as too little oxygen, poor nutrition or fluid intake, medications, or infections. The following material offers suggestions on dealing with patients who have experienced a loss of hearing or eyesight, who have speech disorders, or are confused or disoriented.

Communicating with Hearing-Impaired Patients

The following guidelines can be used.

1. Determine if the patient is using any hearing aids. Then face the patient directly (and on the same level if possible). Use facial expression, body gestures, and touch to add to your communication.
2. Speak in a normal fashion without shouting. Be sure that the light is not shining in the eyes of a patient who is trying to read lips.
3. Reduce background noises when carrying on conversations with the hard-of-hearing patient. Do not eat or chew anything while talking.
4. Be sure to get the patient's attention before you start to speak. Never talk from another room.

5. If the patient has difficulty understanding something, find another way of saying the same thing rather than repeating the original words over and over.

6. Use a pad and pencil whenever necessary. Consider learning sign language as a personal goal if deaf and hard-of-hearing patients constitute a significant portion of your patient population.

Communicating with Visually Impaired Patients

The following guidelines can be used.

1. Determine whether the patient wears any prescribed corrective lenses. Always treat the patient's glasses with care if they must be removed during the examination. To prevent scratches, never place the glass side directly on a hard surface.

2. When ambulating or transferring patients, have them hold onto your arm as you lead the way. Visually impaired patients will sense your movements but must be warned of any steps or hazards.

3. Be sure to use touch and the tone of your voice to help in communicating with the patient.

4. Ask blind patients how they are used to doing things for themselves, and then allow them to continue unless their actions would interfere with their safety.

Communicating with Speech-Impaired Patients

The following guidelines can be used.

1. Encourage patients to express themselves through any means possible. To improve their speaking ability, patients must try to talk, write, and read as much as possible, even if they make mistakes.

2. Keep patients a part of the social world by talking while performing their examination. Encourage your co-workers to do so also.

3. If the patient has difficulty understanding communication, be sure to stand where you can be seen, and speak slowly and clearly in a normal tone of voice. Use common vocabulary and short, simple sentences. Give directions or requests in a simple manner, repeating or rephrasing the directions as necessary. Use simple gestures or pantomime for clarification.

4. For patients who have difficulty speaking, provide ample time for them to organize what they want to say. Do not hurry or pressure them. Watch for clues or gestures if you cannot understand the patient's speech.

5. Be patient. Becoming upset will only add to your patient's frustration. Assist patients with words they cannot say, but do not speak for them. Give them a chance to try to say the words.
6. Do not treat patients as children. Respect them as the adults they are.
7. Use supportive communication (verbal or nonverbal) to help patients handle the frustration and anxiety that they may feel.
8. Never speak with another sonographer or staff member in front of patients as if they were not there just because you think the patient will not understand.

Communicating with Confused or Disoriented Patients

The following guidelines can be used.

1. It is important to keep talking to confused patients. Do not label them confused and then ignore them.
2. Confusion may be greater at some times than others; therefore it is important to talk with the patients and to communicate acceptance and security by verbal and nonverbal means.
3. Listen and try to understand what patients are trying to tell you.
4. Use reality orientation to help patients interact with the world around them. Such techniques are based on sensory stimulation by identifying what is happening around them and clarifying who they are (examples: time of day, day of the week).
5. Keep the environment calm to avoid overwhelming the patient with too many people or too much confusion.
6. Talk face-to-face with the patient, using short, simple sentences. Ask only one question (or give one direction) at a time, and allow ample time for a response. Try to keep the patient looking at you. Be sure to clarify what is happening.
7. Praise and encourage patients in what they are able to do. Encourage as much independence as possible to help them feel better about themselves.
8. Use supportive conversation to help patients when they get frustrated, anxious, or depressed. A gentle, caring attitude will help support the patient during periods of extreme confusion.
9. Remember that patients in restraints may become confused if they cannot interact with their surroundings.
10. Provide the patient with correct information. Do not support patients' confused beliefs or behavior. Correct them gently, however, with supportive communication, and do not argue with patients who continue to be confused.

THE GRIEVING PROCESS

Each of us knows that eventually we are going to die. Obviously, we all have different views about death, based on our backgrounds, past experiences, and religious beliefs. As a sonographer you will come in contact with dying patients or those in danger of losing a pregnancy; thus it is important to explore your feelings about death to better understand your patients' feelings (Craig, 1987a).

The grieving process has been defined as stages of behavior that people experience when a loss occurs. Elisabeth Kübler-Ross, a Swiss-born physician, worked extensively with dying patients and describes the following stages of grief:

Stage 1   Denial and isolation
Stage 2   Anger
Stage 3   Bargaining
Stage 4   Depression
Stage 5   Acceptance

The grieving process often can take a considerable period of time, and passage through it may not always go smoothly or in the "proper" order. Some persons do not experience each stage and may skip one, whereas others may go through more than one stage at a time. Some patients will move back and forth between the stages, feeling that the pain and stress will never go away. Regardless of the individual patient's reaction, it is important that the sonographer treat each one in a supportive manner, with dignity and compassion.

Denial and isolation

The denial or isolation stage occurs for all patients. It is characterized by the "No, not me — it must be some mistake" attitude. The person believes that a diagnostic error has been made and will seek other opinions. The refusal to believe this is happening creates a buffer, protecting the individual from shocking news that is too difficult to handle. Denial provides time for people to collect themselves and to prepare their resources.

Some patients may isolate themselves from those who will not allow them to deny the seriousness of their illness, whereas others try to hide their feelings of sadness or fear by assuming a false front or cheerful attitude. Mood swings from high hopes to despair prevail. One reaction is their need to talk about and explain what has happened — making up excuses and reasons for their loss or illness, but not really believing it. Sonographers should encourage these patients to talk about their feelings — to allow denial of reality and isolation. It is helpful to identify a supportive family member to be present during the patient examinations and transfers. Because denial or repression is a defense mechanism, you must be sure that you have fully assessed the patient's condition and carefully thought out your approach before engaging the patient in conversation.

Anger

This "why me?" stage is difficult for everyone to deal with because of the tendency to displace anger in all directions. Patients at this stage make unreasonable demands or levy unjust criticism at everyone participating in their care. Blaming those around them (family, friends, hospital staff) for their condition, they may be dissatisfied with everything you do. In these ways they are able to express their feelings of losing control over their lives. It is essential to remain patient and try to be understanding by allowing the patient to "act out" feelings. This is not the time to try to divert the patient with humor or cheerfulness. It is a time to carefully explain the nature of the sonographic procedure to avoid patient fear or suspicion. If patients at this stage are given extra attention and a chance to verbalize or act out their anger, they soon become more reasonable and have fewer angry demands.

Another reaction is for patients to display paranoid feelings that staff members are against them or want to hurt them. It is important not to react as if the patient is personally attacking you. Simply understand that through this behavior patients are able to unload the intense and often painful feelings they are experiencing.

Bargaining

As patients begin to accept their condition, they may try to bargain with God—attempting to postpone the inevitable. They may want to be rewarded for good behavior by having special favors granted, or they cling to life until a special event has been experienced. It is in this state of mind that patients desperately try alternative or "quack" treatments. Sonographers should allow such patients to talk about their bargains with God and should share the patient's requests and actions with staff members.

Depression

Depression is encountered when patients finally realize the reality of their loss. Overwhelming sadness and sorrow usually occurs, causing patients to cry, lose interest in their surroundings, and become silent and withdrawn.

Let these patients express sorrow and feel sad. Encouragement and reassurance do not help patients at this stage, and cheerfulness will only distract them and cut off their feelings. Be willing to sit quietly, encouraging the patient to talk about his or her feelings and expressing your own feelings with words of empathy or a simple, caring touch.

Acceptance

With the stage of acceptance, patients are at peace once more and thinking more clearly. Although patients still may not understand the reasons for their condition or believe that they should die, they may want to talk about dying and ask you questions.

This is not a joyful stage. It is instead a controlled stage in which intense feelings are absent. Energy and interest will decrease, and the patient will need the support and company of family and friends. At this point patients need to be told that it is all right to say nothing, to "just be." Appropriate physical touching may replace mere words, so be willing to sit quietly with patients at this stage and to hold their hand or stroke their hair.

Throughout all the stages, the belief that things can get better exists. Hope helps maintain patients through their suffering, and patients should be encouraged to have hope even if it seems unrealistic at times.

Dealing with patients who ask if they are dying is one of the most difficult things for health professionals to handle. Although you may not know the answer to the question or even what the patient has been told, you must resist the temptation to change the subject or tell the patient not to worry. Your answers to questions about dying should be, "What makes you say that?" or "Did your doctor tell you that?" It is simply not your responsibility to tell patients that they are dying or to give them factual information that you have gleaned from their chart or the nursing staff. Acknowledge that such fears are upsetting. Then, after providing a chance to talk, ask if the patient would like to speak with his or her physician or nurse because you do not have additional information. Be sure to report the person's concerns and requests. Above all else, do not leave the patient alone with no one to talk to (Kübler-Ross, 1975).

PROFESSIONAL COMMUNICATION

Communicating with Health Care Co-Workers

Among the communications that are vital to patient/interdepartmental interaction are the following:

- Participation in team conferences, grand rounds, in-service training, departmental meetings
- Interviewing patients
- Instructing patients and their families
- Reporting the patient's sonographic findings to other members of the health care team
- Recording information in daily logs, charts, files

Whether you are a hospital-based or office-based sonographer, you often will be asked to communicate by telephone. When doing so, be sure to give your name and department identification, and also ask for the same information from the calling or called party.

Calls should be answered promptly. This is especially important in the health care arena, where the next call might be an emergency call.

Good telephone etiquette should always be observed. Take messages properly and deliver them promptly. Never cover the receiver and continue a conversation with someone else. Callers usually can hear what is being said.

When asked to schedule patients, be polite, and thoroughly explain any necessary patient preparations. Be fair in awarding the patient the first possible opening, and be accommodating if other tests or treatments conflict with the selected appointment time.

Sonographer Reports

To contribute to the patient's diagnosis in a professional way, sonographers often are asked to provide written or verbal reports. As trained observers of the interaction of ultrasound transmission and reflection characteristics within the human body, sonographers should be prepared to discuss their technical findings. When properly used, sonographer reports serve as aids to diagnosis by documenting normal measurements and by drawing attention to any unusual findings that might indicate the presence of disease and a need for additional examination.

Sonographer reports should be limited to providing measurements, comments on the echogenicity and location of normal and abnormal structures, and any unusual patient positions, scanning planes, or changes in instrumentation that were required to complete the examination.

The use of written sonographer "impressions" is especially warranted in situations in which the interpretation of the sonographic examinations occurs without the sonographer's presence (e.g., after normal hours or in a distant locale). One of the values of recording these impressions is the availability of written documentation in the event that a case is ever questioned. Sonographer reports also serve a teaching function when follow-up data about the patient's final diagnosis and treatment are obtained and compared against the sonography findings.

Unfortunately, there also are negative aspects regarding sonographer reports. There is a real possibility that these technical impressions may be construed as diagnostic statements. This usually happens when the referring physician demands an instant "diagnosis" or preliminary report instead of waiting for the interpreting physician's findings. The potential for abuse also exists if the sonographer's impressions are used verbatim by physicians with little or no training in the interpretation of sonographic images. In addition, serious ethical and legal implications surround the practice of sonographers communicating their impressions directly to the patient or the patient's family (Craig, 1987).

To retain the advantages and to minimize the negative aspects of sonographer reports, the ultrasound facility should draw up and publish policies to guide its sonographers in these situations. These policies should establish exactly what type of information (such as gender identification, estimated fetal age, number of fetuses, fetal viability) sonographers are permitted to disclose and to whom (referring physicians, patients, or family members) the disclosures may be made. The facility should then alert all house staff members and referring physicians to the new policies and the reasons validating their adoption (Craig, 1991).

Videotaping Obstetric Examinations

One of the most controversial sonographic issues is the practice of providing patients with videotapes or Polaroid images of fetal ultrasound examinations or Polaroid images of their fetus. Just as ultrasound has become more technologically sophisticated, so too have the patients in their appreciation and understanding of imaging devices and the content of sonograms (Craig, 1986).

Proponents of videotaping for family members are quick to point out that this practice enhances fetal bonding, educates both patients and family members, and increases patient acceptance of sonography. Those who are opposed to providing images for patient use believe that the practice extends scanning time and patient exposure and, more important, that it distracts the sonographer's concentration and teeters on the brink of commercialization (Craig, 1988).

If videotapes of obstetric examinations are provided to patients in your institution, the following recommendations should be considered.

- A written policy should be established for providing patients with hard-copy images of their sonography examination.
- A specific time should be set aside to create a tape for the patient's use. Preferably, this should take place after completion of the diagnostic examination.
- Nothing should appear on the patient's photographs or tape that was not seen on the diagnostic study or survey.
- The supervising physician must be aware of the examination results and should review the patient's photographs or videotape before they are released to the patient. The physician should exercise the right to deny the tape or photographs for patient use if any abnormality is found or suspected.

SUMMARY

Sonographers can have a profound impact on the patients entrusted to their care. By proper communication techniques they can gain a patient's confidence and cooperation. How they handle their responsibilities can have a direct bearing on the patient's journey to recovery or the patient's lack of progress.

At issue are the positive and negative aspects of patient and interdepartmental communications, as well as some of the perplexing issues involving sonographer reports and possible solutions to those issues.

REFERENCES

Craig, M.: Family-centered sonography. Journal of Diagnostic Medical Sonography 1986;2:96-103.

Craig, M.: The challenge of patient interaction. Journal of Diagnostic Medical Sonography 1987a;3:147-150.

Craig, M.: The eternal controversy: Sonographer's reports. Journal of Diagnostic Medical Sonography 1987b;3:244-248.

Craig, M.: Baby videos: A boon or a liability? Journal of Diagnostic Medical Sonography 1988;4:19-22.

Craig, M.: Treating patients with patience. Journal of Diagnostic Medical Sonography 1989;1:16-18.

Craig, M.: Controversies in obstetric and gynecologic ultrasound. In Diagnostic Medical Sonography: A Guide to Clinical Practice. Vol. 1: Obstetrics and Gynecology. Philadelphia: J. B. Lippincott Co., 1991.

Kübler-Ross, E.: Death: The Final Stage of Growth. Englewood Cliffs, N.J.: Prentice-Hall, 1975.

▼

U N I T 6

Ethics and Professionalism

LEARNING OBJECTIVES

Students who successfully complete this unit will be able to:

- List five basic physiologic needs.
- Describe Maslow's hierarchy of needs.
- Describe the sonographer's role in relation to medical ethics.
- Describe what is meant by professionalism.
- Interact with patients, peers, and other health professionals in a considerate and professional manner.
- Discuss the importance of professional confidentiality.
- Discuss the personal obligations sonographers have to their patients, to other health professionals, and to their profession.
- Define the term *tort* and cite examples that might involve sonographers.
- Discuss the three forms of patient consent.
- Define the doctrines of *respondeat superior* and *res ipsa locquitur* and explain how they may apply to sonographers and sonography services.
- Discuss the common reasons a sonographer may be named defendant in a malpractice case.
- Discuss the recommended steps sonographers should take to protect themselves against malpractice suits.

For many years the health care profession was governed by rigid, no-nonsense rules that discouraged any emotional or personal involvement with patients, and it demanded unquestioning obedience to authority figures. The training of health care practitioners in the past was limited to specialized classes devoted to the recognition of normal and abnormal body structure and functions and the techniques of meeting the physiologic needs of such patients. Classroom theories were reinforced by countless hours of practical, voluntary, on-the-job training.

As the various health professions evolved during the second half of this century, academic programs were incorporated into the training process and concern for the psychosocial aspects of health care began to emerge. Courses in the behavioral sciences of psychology and sociology were added to curricula in the hope that the knowledge of theory in these areas would improve graduates' ability to understand and cope with the personal problems of their patients.

Little effort, however, was made to relate these new curriculum components to the practical rules that governed the conduct and performance of the health care professional. As a result, the two varieties of professional instruction coexisted without any basic integration (Purtilo, 1984).

For the past four decades the arbitrary rules that governed the professions have been challenged and, in some cases, rejected. Studies in the behavioral sciences have been expanded, but, more important, the health specialties have begun to build bridges between theory and patient interaction.

Formerly rigid professional-role behaviors have become more sensible and flexible. An integrated focus of helping patients get well, as well as tolerate and reduce the psychologic discomfort of their illnesses, has elevated the patient from being a "case" to being a person. In this discovery process, health care practitioners have begun to analyze their own psychosocial conditions as they strive to become the best they can be. The goal of this unit is to explore these needs, as well as the aspirations of all people, as a means to improving the quality of life.

BASIC HUMAN NEEDS

If life is to be sustained, certain basic survival needs must be met. Food, water, and oxygen are the most critical; other physiologic needs include rest and sleep, elimination of waste products, activity and exercise, shelter, and sexual needs.

According to the work of Carl Rogers and A. H. Maslow, once the basic biologic needs of water, food, sleep, sex, and so on, have been provided, human beings develop complex emotional needs (Feldman, 1990; Maslow, 1987; Rogers, 1977). Maslow called them a *hierarchy of needs*. Ascending from the basic biologic needs to complex psychosocial motivations, these secondary needs are vital to preserving the quality of life.

Like steppingstones, each need must be fulfilled before an individual is comfortable and secure enough to move on to the other, or next, needs. Maslow defined these secondary needs as security, belonging and acceptance, self-esteem, and self-actualization.

The highest motive is self-actualization, a state of self-fulfillment that allows one to reach his or her full potential. However, self-actualization can be achieved only after all the other needs have been met. By studying men and women who had made extraordinary use of their potential, Maslow arrived at a composite picture of self-actualizers and the distinguishing characteristics of such persons: well-balanced, perceptive, honest, independent, creative, caring, and courageous. The implications of Maslow's theories are significant; by understanding the hierarchy of needs, health care professionals can reach their primary goal of helping patients who are unable to meet their own needs because of illness, injury, or aging.

ETHICS

In general terms, *ethics* can be described as the disciplined study of morality as it concerns conduct and character. *Medical ethics* grows out of the patient-physician relationship and mandates that physicians know what is in the best interest of their patients, and that they "do no harm" (Beauchamp and Childress, 1989).

Sonographers, acting under the direction of physicians, share these ethical obligations to protect and promote the best interests of their patients. Working together, sonologists and sonographers cooperatively seek a correct diagnosis through the use of high-frequency ultrasound imaging.

The ethics of sonography can currently be analyzed only in terms of the sonographer's role as a member of the health care team. This situation exists because sonography is an emerging, but not yet fully autonomous, profession. Chervenak and McCullough (1991) cite social workers as an example of health professionals who have achieved autonomy by developing patient-client categories (e.g., the dysfunctional family, the victims of child abuse).

At the present time, sonography lacks any method of establishing reliable diagnostic categories and nomenclature that is independent of physicians. Thus, until sonographers possess full autonomy, they will be limited to performing as agents of the physician.

Since the second half of the twentieth century, patients have formulated their own ideas about their best interests and have developed the capacity to express and carry out value-based preferences. They have achieved patient autonomy and, in doing so, have obligated health professionals to acknowledge their values and beliefs and to avoid interfering with their expression or implementation.

Obstetric Issues

More than any other sonographic specialty, obstetrics has produced difficult ethical questions and dilemmas. An obstetric sonographer must serve two patients—mother and fetus—even though the obligations to both parties sometimes seem at cross-purposes. The concept of a fetus as a patient in need of consideration, care, and sometimes corrective protection has been widely accepted (Heintze, 1987).

In pregnancies that progress to term, sonographers are expected to provide clinical protection and promotion of fetal interests, because fetuses are not autonomous. Through their imaging skills, sonographers contribute to the prevention of premature death, disease, handicapping conditions, and unnecessary pain and suffering. These obligations do not extend, however, to previable fetuses that are aborted (Chervenak and McCullough, 1985; 1989).

The failure of society to achieve emotional resolution and political clarity regarding the sanctity of life with regard to abortion or selective fetal termination has created a tenuous legal, ethical, and moral climate (Weiss, 1985). As a result, sonographers must be very aware of the assertion of fetal rights—aware that they are legally responsible for their actions and diagnosis until the fetal patient reaches the age of majority (Craig, 1991).

Some sonographers may have moral objections to abortion. If so, they should approach the request for their services by avoiding moral judgment of the pregnant woman and respecting her autonomy, realizing that the patient and her physician have considered her problems and have based their decision on multiple factors that may be unknown to the sonographer. Regardless of personal beliefs, it is not the province of sonographers to attempt to dissuade, encourage, or punish their patients. Instead, sonographers should take a personal inventory of their feelings and beliefs regarding abortion and medical intervention procedures. Those unable to accept the current laws and medical practices regarding them must express their convictions to their supervisors and request to be relieved of the duty of working with patients destined to undergo such procedures. The sonographer's beliefs also must be respected, and there should be no fear of professional or economic reprisals. Once a sonographer accepts responsibility toward a patient, however, he or she must never refuse to carry out or complete a procedure (Craig, 1991).

Confidentiality

Another ethical concern is that of confidentiality. Sonographers, physicians, and patients compose the three personal elements of medical sonography examinations. Diagnostic information about a patient therefore can be justifiably disclosed to outside parties *only with the patient's approval and explicit permission.*

Competency

As a sonographer, you will have a basic ethical obligation to perform a competent examination and to provide physicians and patients with accurate and reliable information. It requires continuing education, as well as preparatory training, to ensure that you maintain a general level of competence in sonography. A serious breach of ethics results whenever sonographers lag behind the advances made in their field. By performing inaccurate or incomplete examinations, or reporting the results of such examinations to patients, they undermine the physician's trust and reliance on sonographers.

If sonographers discover errors based on faulty equipment, technique, or interpretation, they have a duty to bring such errors to the attention of the interpreting physician. Sonographers can be placed in an adverse position if the errors are not corrected or communicated by the interpreting physician to the referring physician. Then, as patient advocates, sonographers must express their concerns *directly* to the referring physician and, in some cases, also may be required to disclose such information to the pregnant woman (Chervenak and McCullough, 1991).

Although sonographers have serious ethical obligations, they do not enjoy unlimited freedom because their roles are derived from the patient-physician relationship. This factor, in addition to sonography's evolutionary quality, creates some degree of difficulty in practicing ethical distinctions. Nevertheless, these distinctions are crucial to provide an understanding of the sonographer's proper role in the health care team. Toward that goal, it is extremely important that internal policies and procedures reflecting the ethical concerns raised in this unit should be defined, drafted, and implemented by sonographers and their supervising physicians. Only in this way will sonographers be able to discharge their duties without evading their responsibilities or breaking the patient's trust.

PROFESSIONALISM

There is considerable overlap in the topics of ethics and professionalism, and to many, the terms are synonymous. Professionalism in health care is based on integrity and honesty as well as compassion. The ethics of our profession also demand that conduct toward patients be totally devoid of any self-interest. It is for this reason that in addition to developing technical knowledge and skills, sonographers also must learn about the standards and the conduct that are expected of them.

A *professional* is a person who does something with great skill and who meets the high standards of his or her profession.

The key to developing professionalism is understanding. Professional sonographers are sonographers who understand what their job is, which enables them to direct their energies toward performing that job. The "pros" also understand the roles of other people in their profession—patients, physicians, and a wide variety of health specialists—and have acquired the ability to deal with each other in terms of reasonable expectations. Experience provides this understanding; however, experience takes time.

If you wish to be thought of as a professional, you must be willing to ask for information and guidance, to seek explanations of terms and jargon, to become skillful at interacting with your patients, and to learn how clinicians think in order to develop a dialogue with them and their agents. You also will need to understand and inform those within your professional sphere not only about the strengths but about the limitations of sonography and its purveyors.

Interactions with Patients

The primary attribute of health professionals is their inseparable identification with human suffering. Their concern carries with it feelings of responsibility for patients and a willingness to serve all of the sick and helpless entrusted to their care (Purtilo, 1984).

Patients usually come to the sonographer for diagnostic assistance because of the presence of some symptom (e.g., pain, disability, questions involving pregnancy). In most instances the patient-sonographer relationship is over when the examination is completed and the patient leaves the sonography department. During the time patients are with sonographers, however, they may need reassurance about their physical problems and understanding and guidance to help them adjust to their new situation.

You must consider carefully not only what to say to your patients but also how to deliver the information. Keep in mind that patients often do not fully understand what is said, or they may misunderstand or take statements out of context. Some patients hear only what they wish to hear! Nevertheless, do not let these factors deter you from communicating with your patients, because such communication can be one of the most rewarding experiences available to you. Instead, work toward preparing your patients psychologically for their examinations by explaining the procedure and establishing realistic expectations (Craig, 1989; Lea, 1985).

Avoiding Dehumanization

Each patient brings some degree of anxiety to the examination. Each one is concerned with how this illness will affect daily life, loved ones, and activities.

Too often, health practitioners think of patients in the abstract terms of their condition *(Is the gallbladder in Room 3?)*. You must avoid that kind of trap and always accord your patients respect for their individuality as well as their physical condition.

Sonographer Competence

Patients arrive at their sonography examination with very clear expectations of the person who will be conducting their examination, and they respond according to the treatment they receive. For instance, some patients may refuse to submit to an examination by a "student," simply because they perceive a student as someone who is not yet fully trained or competent. Observing the interaction of sonographers with their co-workers and other health professionals also can influence a patient's perceptions of professionalism. Patients have little confidence in sonographers who exhibit overly casual or immature behavior.

In addition to expectations of professional conduct, patients expect sonographers to project a professional image. Specific standards of dress and grooming must be met because patients' first impressions are strongly influenced by personal appearance. The dress and grooming of the entire staff and the appearance of the sonography section and the institution that houses it can influence patient opinions. Neatness, cleanliness, and friendly efficiency are essential to inspire patient confidence.

Although social attitudes, dress, and grooming have become more casual, nothing changes the fact that *casualness* does not epitomize the *professional image* of health care personnel that has been perpetuated in the mind of the public for many years. Each hospital, clinic, or ultrasound practice establishes appropriate dress and grooming codes to reflect its professionalism. Sonographers must adhere to these guidelines or regulations regardless of their own personal taste.

Recognizing Transference

The act of shifting one's feelings about a person in the past to another person is called *transference*. Both negative and positive reactions can be stimulated, such as feelings of hostility, cooperation, and confidence (Purtilo, 1984). Thus sonographers must conduct themselves properly during all patient interactions, communicating concern yet maintaining a professional distance. They must respect and give service with equal care and dedication to all patients regardless of sex, race, creed, color, or economic background.

Protecting Patient Modesty

One particularly sensitive area of interaction is consideration for the patient's modesty. By observing the rules of draping and covering the patient to the greatest extent possible during an examination, sonographers can reduce patient anxiety. Providing privacy when patients disrobe or perform bodily functions will be appreciated by most patients and will obtain their grateful cooperation. When examinations require patients to be exposed or to assume positions that are potentially embarrassing, sonographers must use considerable tact to preserve the patient's modesty and personal dignity, even if it means stepping aside in favor of a sonographer who is of the same sex as the patient.

Interacting with Difficult Patients

Professionals learn to master verbal communication, facial expression, and other facets of body language. They learn to converse intelligently, pleasantly, and courteously with patients. If a patient is under stress or is unpleasant to deal with, a professional is able to maintain emotional control and attempts to alleviate the patient's apprehension and to determine what is causing the unpleasant behavior.

During their initial contact with patients, sonographers are expected to determine the most appropriate manner in which to deal with a particular patient. They should communicate their interest in the patient at all times and provide assurance at the end of the examination that they have given their best services.

Confidentiality

Professional confidentiality imposes a major restriction on the health professional. Because medical and personal patient information must always be held in strict confidence, revealing such data to patients, family, or others outside the department cannot occur without the direct consent of the patient's physician. Failure to respect the patient's rights in this regard can result in legal problems.

Interacting with Other Health Professionals

As a student and ultimately as a graduate sonographer, you will be required to interact with many different health professionals. Initially your time is spent with your instructors. These often are professional sonographers who have developed the teaching skills necessary to prepare you academically and technically for the role of the sonographer. Instructors also can offer the benefit of their personal experience to ease their students' entry into the patient setting and to help them develop professional judgment.

Although most physicians, nurses, and other health workers will be friendly and cooperative, you may find some who seem distant, preoccupied, or indifferent. In many instances this negative behavior is the result of an ongoing and wide gap in professional standing between the medical and the technical fields. Rather than becoming part of such a problem, a professional will find ways to break the cycle. By asking for guidance or information from physicians or by expressing an interest in how other departments function and what ideas they might have improving interdepartmental cooperation, effective bridges can be created to span such gaps.

Obligations toward the Sonography Profession

Your first obligation to sonography is to recognize that it is more than just a job. This realization should motivate you not only to become proficient but to continue to grow with the field so that you do not become "second rate."

In addition to pursuing continuing education, you should participate in and support the activities of your professional organizations. Many offer student membership categories and special services that can help you master the skills you desire. The universal benefits of

Table 6–1. Code of Professional Conduct for Diagnostic Medical Sonographers

Preamble

The Code of Professional Conduct of the Society of Diagnostic Medical Sonographers is a statement of the high standards of conduct toward which sonographers are committed to strive. Sonographers, as members of a health care profession, acknowledge their responsibilities to their patients, to other health care professionals, and to each other.

   I. **Sonographers** shall act in the best interest of the patient.

  II. **Sonographers** shall provide sonographic services with compassion, respect for human dignity, honesty, and integrity.

 III. **Sonographers** shall respect the patient's right to privacy, safeguarding confidential information within the constraints of the law.

 IV. **Sonographers** shall maintain competence in their field.

  V. **Sonographers** shall assume responsibility for their actions.

Reprinted with permission from the Society of Diagnostic Medical Sonographers.

membership in such groups include resources that provide the following advantages:

- Helping maintain high educational and performance standards
- Advancing professional stature
- Providing a training ground for leadership applicable to your laboratory, your institution, and your profession

Your ultimate obligation to your profession is to pursue excellence and superior performance. Through the efforts of the Society of Diagnostic Medical Sonographers, a code of conduct for sonographers has been developed (Table 6–1).

MEDICOLEGAL CONSIDERATIONS

Laws are the rules of conduct recognized by custom or formal enactment, which a community considers binding upon its members. Medical law deals with a particular sphere of human activity—the care of the patient. It is the goal of medical law to protect people, to correct injustice, and to compensate for injury.

Along with the permission to practice medicine, society demands that physicians conduct their practices according to accepted standards. Any failure to adequately meet these codes of conduct leaves the physician *and his or her agents* open to civil actions.

Laws that govern individual rights in noncriminal actions are called *torts,* "a wrongful act, injury, or damage (not involving a breach of contract), for which a civil action can be brought" (Webster, 2nd college ed.). There are two types of torts: those that result from intentional action and those that result from unintentional action. It is important to note that civil wrongs also can be crimes.

The following section notes several situations in which tort action can be taken against health professionals because of their deliberate actions (Gurley and Calloway, 1986).

Intentional Misconduct

Assault, battery, invasion of privacy, and false imprisonment are some types of intentional misconduct.

Assault

The threat or unsuccessful attempt to injure another in an illegal manner, causing present fear of immediate harm, is considered assault.

Example. Any sonographer who indulges in imprudent conduct, causing a patient to be apprehensive of injury, could be held liable or responsible to provide financial compensation to the patient for damages that may have resulted from the apprehension.

Battery

Battery is the unlawful touching of another person directly or with an object, without that person's consent, with or without resultant injury. Assault and battery often are charged together because of a successful attempt to injure.

Example. Sonographers cannot touch patients for any reason unless there is a valid consent by the patient to receive medical care. If any bodily harm has been inflicted on a patient, the potential for liability against the sonographer exists.

Invasion of privacy

This is the wrongful intrusion into another person's private activities, which causes humiliation or mental suffering or unlawfully makes public any knowledge concerning private or personal information without the consent of the wronged person.

Example. A sonographer who publicly discusses privileged and confidential information obtained from the attending physician or the patient's medical record can be sued for invasion of privacy.

False imprisonment

This is the holding or detaining of a person against his or her will.

Example. Sonographers could be charged with false imprisonment if they unnecessarily confine or restrain a patient without obtaining permission from the patient to be so restricted.

Other forms

Other forms of intentional misconduct include spoken *(slander)* or written *(libel)* defamation.

Unintentional Misconduct-Negligence

Negligence is the failure to perform in a reasonably prudent manner or to fulfill the expected standards of care.

Example. Any sonographer who unintentionally causes injury to a patient may be accused of committing a negligent act. If a sonographer who intended to help actually caused damage by failure to perform as the patient and the employer had the right to expect, a tort action may be brought by either the patient or the employer. To establish negligence and culpability for damages in court, the civil proceedings must address the issues of duty, breach, cause, and injury.

Duty. This relates to the *standard of care.* A sonographer is obliged under law to perform services for a patient that meet current national standards of practice.

Breach. Breach is failure of a sonographer to exercise reasonable care, resulting in patient injury *(this could be interpreted to include failure of the sonographer to produce a scan with adequate diagnostic information).*

Cause. Cause is injury resulting as a direct cause of the sonographer's negligence (e.g., failure to raise side rails before leaving an incapacitated patient unattended).

Injury. Any hurt a patient sustains as a result of sonographer negligence.

Consent

Consent can be defined as *permission granted voluntarily by a person in his or her right mind.* Patients have the right to consent to or refuse any service of a hospital or other medical setting. Such consent can be written, oral, or implied. Consent is valid only if the patient (1) is of legal age, (2) is mentally competent, (3) gives consent voluntarily, and (4) is adequately informed about the medical care being recommended (i.e., understands the type of care and potential risks).

The sonographer should be aware of the following considerations.

1. Written consent is favored because it is easier to prove (Fig. 6–1).
2. Implied consent (usually used when an unconscious patient is at risk) assumes that the patient would want consent extended to secure care.
3. Patients can revoke consent at any time — whether or not previous verbal, written, or implied consent was given by the patient. At no time can that patient be *denied the right* to withdraw or revoke consent.

Respondeat Superior

The doctrine of *respondeat superior requires that an employer* pay the victim for the torts against the employee. This Latin phrase can be translated literally as *"Let the master answer"* (Gurley and Callaway, 1986). This means that hospitals or physicians who employ a sonographer can be held jointly responsible for whatever the sonographer did in a negligent manner. Injured patients are not required to prove that the *employer* was negligent, only that the *sonographer* was liable.

Although hospital or physician employers may automatically be held jointly liable, sonographers are not necessarily immune from damage suits nor in any way relieved of personal responsibility for breach of duty. Because all persons are responsible for their own injurious conduct, the employer may opt to bring suit against the sonographer.

Res Ipsa Loquitur

In some cases of negligence, defendants are required to prove innocence. The Latin phrase *res ipsa loquitur* means "the thing speaks for itself." It is necessary for the defendant to demonstrate that injury could not have occurred if there had been no negligence and that the defendant was in no way responsible for the negligent act (Gurley and Calloway, 1986).

Protection Against Lawsuits

Although sonographers generally work under the direction of a physician, they are still personally liable for any harm a patient suffers as a result of their own acts.

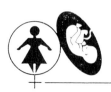

FRANKLIN MEDICAL ASSOCIATES, P.C.
OBSTETRICS/GYNECOLOGY/INFERTILITY
(313) 353-0100

A. Lewis Hayes, M.D. / Michael S. Salesin, M.D. / Alan D. Goldsmith, M.D.

26206 West Twelve Mile Road / Suite 200 / Southfield, Michigan 48034

INFORMED CONSENT FOR INTRAVAGINAL ULTRASOUND

Intravaginal ultrasound is a technique where the ultrasound transducer (sensing unit) is placed in the vagina rather than other techniques where the unit is placed on the patient's abdomen. This technique is used when there are specific indications which require this kind of results. These indications include very early pregnancy, use of infertility drugs and concern over ovarian disease.

I/We, the undersigned, have agreed to allow Dr. _____ to perform an intravaginal ultrasound examination. This examination is performed using the vaginal approach to gain additional information versus that obtained from a transabdominal study.

Although intravaginal ultrasound is a technique which has been used extensively and so far no hazards have been discovered, it cannot be guaranteed that the procedure will not cause damage to the patient nor to a fetus if the patient is pregnant. In the case of a pregnancy, it cannot be guaranteed that the procedure will not initiate a miscarriage.

Signed:

_____
Patient

_____
Husband/Parent/Significant Other

_____
Witness

_____
Date

Figure 6–1. Example of a current informed consent form. *(Courtesy Michael S. Salesin, M.D.)*

Legal actions involving negligence by a person engaged in a profession are generally known as *malpractice* suits. Many professionals protect themselves from such possible legal actions by carrying malpractice insurance obtained through private insurance companies or through professional organizations. Such policies should cover legal fees and judgment expenses in the event that the sonographer is sued for malpractice. In addition, the term of coverage must adequately protect obstetric sonographers who are later sued by individuals who were *fetal* patients at the time of the alleged negligence or malpractice. However, it should be noted that some professionals feel that lawyers target individuals with coverage.

Sonographers should understand that even if they are innocent of charges, it will still cost them money to prepare a defense, as well as lost wages because of time spent in court.

We expect malpractice insurance to cover any charges brought against sonographers, providing the sonographers have practiced within the limits of their job description and level of training. The sonographer should consider the following important guidelines.

- Always perform procedures as taught or as outlined in the procedures manual of your laboratory or health facility. If such policies are outmoded or incorrect, work through proper channels to improve them.
- Remember, you are responsible for your own behavior. Therefore, refuse to perform procedures for which you have not been prepared. Ignorance is not a legal defense any more than lack of sleep or overwork are acceptable legal reasons for carelessness or mistakes.
- Ask for assistance when you are not sure how to perform a procedure. Do not assume responsibilities beyond your level of knowledge. It would be better to admit that you do not know how to do something than to attempt to do it and bring harm to the patient.
- Keep exact records of all procedures—your technical impressions as well as the physicians' findings. Record any unusual patient behavior or incidents that might have occurred while the patient was in your care. Records of studies involving pregnancy and fetuses should be kept for longer periods (until the fetal patient reaches the age of majority) than are other types of patient studies.
- Learn what legal protection you are provided by your employer, as well as the terms of employment in relation to duties and salary.
- Determine if there are any licensing laws in the state in which you practice. Because malpractice laws vary from state to state, also

review the medical malpractice laws in effect in the state in which you are employed. Determine if any of your work practices place you in violation of those laws.

SUMMARY

The expanding role of diagnostic ultrasound has had a profound impact on medicine and has resulted in many revolutionary changes in patient evaluation and treatment. It has also simultaneously raised some ethical questions.

The best testimonial sonographers can offer their profession is found in daily interactions that result in a patient who has been served well, treated fairly, and received the sonographer's personal best. If you wish to reach these goals, you must apply your knowledge and training in sonography to perform in the following manner.

Do:

- Thoroughly explain the procedure and what you expect of the patient.
- Work with extreme care to avoid causing the patient injury.
- Question any abnormal instructions.
- Maintain records and documents of the procedures you perform in the event you are asked to provide information at a later date.
- Use common sense and judgment, and practice within the limits of your abilities and as you were taught.

Do not:

- Perform sonography procedures that you have not been taught.
- Fail to meet the established standards for the safe care of patients.
- Fail to prevent injury to co-workers, other hospital employees, or visitors, because you may subsequently be sued for damages.

REFERENCES

Beauchamp, T. L., and Childress, J. F.: Principles of Biomedical Ethics, 3rd ed. New York: Oxford University Press, 1989.

Chervenak, F. A., and McCullough, L. B.: Perinatal ethics: A practical analysis of obligations to mother and fetus. Obstetrics and Gynecology 1985;66:442-446.

Chervenak, F. A., and McCullough, L. B.: Ethics in obstetric ultrasound. Journal of Ultrasound in Medicine 1989;8:493-497.

Chervenak, F. A., and McCullough, L. B.: Ethical issues in obstetric sonography. In Berman, M., editor: Diagnostic Medical Sonography: A Guide To Clinical Practice. Vol. 1: Obstetrics and Gynecology. Philadelphia: J. B. Lippincott Co., 1991.

Craig, M.: Treating patients with patience. Journal of Diagnostic Medical Sonography 1989;1:16-18.

Craig, M.: Controversies in obstetric and gynecologic ultrasound. In Berman, M., editor: Diagnostic Medical Sonography: A Guide to Clinical Practice. Vol. 1: Obstetrics and Gynecology. Philadelphia: J. B. Lippincott Co., 1991.

Feldman, R.: Understanding Psychology, 2nd ed. New York: McGraw-Hill, 1990.

Gurley, L. T., and Callaway, W. J.: Introduction To Radiologic Technology, 2nd ed. St. Louis: C. V. Mosby, 1986.

Heintze, C.: Medical Ethics. New York: Franklin Watts Co., 1987.

Lea, J. H.: Psychosocial progression through normal pregnancy. A model for sonographer-patient interaction. Journal of Diagnostic Medical Ultrasound 1985;1:55-58.

Maslow, A. H.: Self-actualization and beyond. In Bugenthal, J. F. T., editor: Challenges of Humanistic Psychology. New York: McGraw-Hill, 1967.

Maslow, A. H.: Motivation and Personality, 2nd ed. New York: Harper & Row, 1987.

Purtilo, R.: Health Professional/Patient Interaction, 3rd ed. Philadelphia: W. B. Saunders Co., 1984.

Rogers, C.: Carl Rogers on Personal Power. New York: Delacorte Press, 1977.

Weiss, A. E.: Bioethics. Dilemmas in Modern Medicine. Hillside, N.J.: Enslow Publishers, Inc., 1985.

▼
─────────────────────────────────

UNIT 7

Environment

LEARNING OBJECTIVES

Students who successfully complete this unit will be able to:

- Compare and contrast the roles and functions of hospitals and clinics.
- Describe the chain of command commonly operating in an imaging department.
- Appreciate the nonimaging roles of the sonographer in relation to referring physicians and other staff members.
- Discuss the major aspects of establishing a sonography service.
- List three common nonhospital sonography settings.
- Describe the similarities and differences of the sonographer's role in hospital and nonhospital settings.

As you near the end of your training experience, you will engage in looking for your first job as a sonographer. Some of you will choose to specialize in a single branch of medical sonography, whereas others who want broader exposure will look for a setting in which they can practice and increase their specialty skills. Hospitals, clinics, office practices, and mobile services are the most common settings for graduate sonographers to begin their careers. This unit explores those settings and their hierarchies and acquaints you with the planning and implementation of a sonographic imaging service.

INSTITUTIONAL SETTINGS

Hospitals

Hospitals are the largest and most common locations of medical imaging services. With a mission to provide treatment and diagnosis both to in-patients and to out-patients, a hospital requires the services of many skilled and unskilled individuals. You, as a newly employed sonographer, will have to become acquainted with and work cooperatively with most of them.

The term *hospital* describes an institution for the reception, medical treatment, and care of the sick or wounded. The original definition of the word derived from the term *hospes,* or guest, and referred to an inn offering hospitality to those in need of shelter and maintenance.

Through the years, hospitals generally have been nonprofit, charitable institutions, often operated by religious groups and generally administered by retired physicians. Today's hospitals still provide for the care of the sick and the wounded, but many are operated as businesses instead of charitable organizations.

Administration. At the top of the chain of command, overseeing all of the hospital activities, is the administrator, or chief executive officer. Surrounding this individual is a large support staff whose task is to administer the daily business affairs of the institution. Your first experience with this administrative staff will likely be with the personnel department. You also will enjoy the services of the accounting department, which issues payroll checks, and if you require personal medical services at any time, you may interact with the insurance and accounts-payable division. The purchasing department of the hospital also falls within the administrative services, and you may work with these employees when you request – or are asked to evaluate – diagnostic ultrasound equipment. As you become a contributing employee of the sonography service, you also may consult or be consulted by the legal representative of the hospital to develop policies and procedures for your department.

Operations. Under this category are all the services necessary to keep the physical plant running, such as maintenance, laundry, central supply, housekeeping, food services, mail room, and communication services. You should visit each of these areas during your new-employee orientation. You will learn firsthand that without the services of these employees there would be no working environment.

Medical staff. The physician component of the medical staff includes the chief physician, staff physicians, residents, fellows, and interns. As a sonographer, you will be called on frequently to communicate with referring physicians and their staff members. Whether scheduling patients or relaying the results of their examinations, you must be knowledgeable, articulate, precise, cooperative, and courteous. You will be expected to follow your department's policies regarding scheduling and the transmission of examination results. You also may be required to assist staff members or referring physicians with procedures such as biopsies, aspirations, amniocentesis, and catheterizations.

Nursing staff. The nursing services administrator usually oversees the operation of the nursing staff. Head or charge nurses and staff nurses—both registered nurses (RNs) and vocational or practical nurses (LVNs/LPNs)—usually constitute the nursing staff. Nurse's aides, orderlies, and ward clerks also report to nursing services.

There are many specialty departments within the hospital, such as pharmacy, surgery, nursery, labor and delivery, and emergency. All, including the imaging department, are organized and operated under a similar chain of command. Sonography services may be part of the radiology department, the nuclear medicine department, noninvasive imaging department, or an adjunct to other departments such as cardiology and obstetrics (Fig. 7–1).

Clinics

A clinic is a smaller version of the hospital, with the exception that it usually does not provide 24-hour or in-patient services. It will have many—but not all—of the professional services offered in a hospital setting. Sonography services may be centralized in an imaging department with the sonography staff expected to perform a broad spectrum of sonography studies. A similar chain of command exists in a clinic setting.

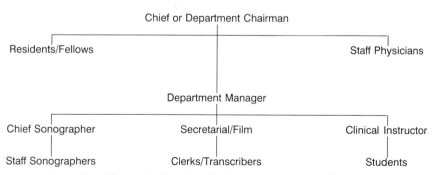

Figure 7–1. Example of an imaging department chain of command.

ESTABLISHING A SONOGRAPHY SERVICE OR LABORATORY

Most sonographers begin their work in an established sonography laboratory. In some instances, however, the sonographer must literally start from scratch. The following recommendations provide a framework for initiating such a project.

Needs assessment. A needs analysis is a prerequisite to designing a sonography laboratory or restructuring (or even understanding) an existing one (Sternlight, 1991). Among the questions to be answered are the following:

- What specific examinations will be performed?
- What types of patients will be examined?
- What kinds of equipment will be required?
- What types of personnel will be required?
- What supplies will be needed?

Budget. A major concern in establishing and implementing an imaging laboratory deals with finances. Drawing up a budget to identify available funds, anticipated operating expenses, and discretionary funding (e.g., continuing education, travel to seminars) will determine the size and scope of the laboratory.

Policies and procedures manual. The drafting of a policies and procedures manual should rank high on your priority list. This type of document should contain the answers to many of the aforementioned questions. It requires input not only from sonographers and sonologists but also from all ancillary personnel whose performance will affect or be affected by such policies. Although this is a major undertaking, the policies and procedures manual will become the definitive reference for all personnel, new and old. Because each laboratory is different, policies and procedures manuals are intended to set guidelines specific to the particular laboratory. Such manuals should cover many diverse items such as job descriptions, scanning protocols, dress codes, interdisciplinary conduct, and emergency procedures. Your manual will quickly become the most valuable and important resource for your laboratory.

Inventory. You will need to create an inventory checklist. Major items, such as ultrasound equipment, clinical supplies (e.g., acoustic coupling media, gloves, masks), and clerical supplies (e.g., requisitions, report forms, stationery, business machines), are obvious; however, personal supplies (such as laboratory coats, calculators, and reference books and charts) also should be included.

Maintenance. Decisions will have to be made regarding laboratory maintenance. General upkeep of cleaning and supplies usually are handled by the housekeeping department. It is vitally important, however, that preventive maintenance be provided for the costly diagnostic ultrasound units. You will need to begin a log that details each piece of equipment. Document all service problems and repairs, indicate terms of any maintenance contracts, and list the names of the sales and service representatives.

Operational procedures such as scanning protocols and the recording and filing of diagnostic images should be developed. Printed forms or instructions should be designed to cover such aspects as patient scheduling, teaching files, and general record keeping.

The ultrasound suite. Space . . . space . . . space! The ultrasound suite should be spacious enough to permit unobstructed traffic flow, with room for expansion or acquisition of additional personnel or equipment. Ample room for maneuvering wheelchairs and stretchers into the scanning area and up to the scanning table is essential. Doorways leading into the facility should be wide enough to admit not only stretchers but patient beds. Consider using bifold doors or sliding-panel door instead of the standard 24- to 36-inch wide doors that are readily available (Craig, 1985). Without adequate room you may be tempted to adapt your movements to the needs of your environment, which might result in assisting patients from a wheelchair or stretcher from an awkward position, increasing the potential for back injuries.

Additional floor space should be available for desks or writing surfaces, linen hampers, and supply cabinets and shelves. To conserve floor space you may wish to have wall-mounted view boxes and telephone systems.

Providing a safe and comfortable working environment for the sonographer and patient is obvious. What is not so obvious is the need to provide the same conditions for the ultrasound equipment. Situate the equipment in such a way that adequate air flow for cooling the instrument is maintained. Ultrasound units are, after all, very sophisticated computers and, like all computers, will function best in a constant room temperature of approximately 70 degrees. The internal temperature of an ultrasound unit that is operating for 4 to 8 hours is double that of the room temperature. Overheating can result in serious degradation of diagnostic images.

The next most important aspect is lighting. It should be variable, from incandescent to fluorescent, with optional rheostat controls.

Any existing windows should be covered with shades, blinds, or drapes to eliminate glare. Scanning is best performed in reduced or low-level lighting so that subtle changes on the oscilloscope screen can quickly be identified.

Because electrical interference occurs so frequently in hospital environments, a dedicated line of power to the ultrasound suite is desirable. Wall outlets—at least one, if not two—should be provided on each wall to reduce the clutter of a tangle of electrical cords and the temptation to plug too many electrical devices into a single outlet.

Bathroom facilities ideally should be located within the ultrasound suite to accommodate the full-bladder patient preparation that so often is part of an ultrasound examination. If this is not feasible, to reduce the chances of infection some hand-washing facility should be available within the laboratory to permit cleansing of the transducers and the sonographer's hands between patient examinations.

These recommendations represent only bare-bones suggestions to get you started if you are given the responsibility of initiating a sonography service. It is a large but not an impossible task. No matter how spacious or well-equipped an ultrasound suite or laboratory is, however, the key to smooth and trouble-free operation lies in following established procedures on a daily basis.

NONHOSPITAL SETTINGS

Office Practices

It is inevitable that technologic advances will be incorporated into physicians' clinical practices. Usually the only limitations are cost and difficulty of operation. As a result, sonographers may find a request for their services in private office settings. Just as the clinic evolved as a smaller version of the hospital, so also does the office practice mirror the clinic in miniature form.

Working as a sonographer in an office practice allows for clinical specialization and the promise of a unique and personalized learning experience.

Depending on the structure of the office hierarchy, the sonographer may work independently or be expected to conform to office policies and procedures. The operational, clinical, and personal inventories will be much smaller, and activities will be limited to examining ambulatory office patients referred by a select group of physicians.

Mobile Ultrasound Services

The most obvious difference between a mobile setting and the more traditional hospital-based or clinic-based laboratory is that the sonographer and equipment must be *absolutely self-sufficient* (Sternlight, 1991).

Mobile ultrasound services may operate in outlying hospitals, clinics, or within the confines of the mobile transport vehicle itself.

Specially adapted and equipped company-owned vans are provided to each sonographer. In addition to traveling to the patients and performing the sonography examinations, mobile sonographers are responsible for equipment and vehicle maintenance (such as gasoline, repairs, and administrative tasks such as keeping track of insurance/warranty policies and telephone pagers), billing clients, maintaining their own time cards, and delivering and/or transmitting their diagnostic images for interpretation if their client hospitals have no qualified physician interpreters on staff.

Mobile sonographers must be exceptionally experienced and particularly independent. Because typically they have no one to consult on questions in their field, their clinical and administrative judgment must be excellent (Sternlight, 1991). They also must be physically fit to transport equipment in and out of the vans at each stop. It is important that they be skilled drivers, experienced in all-weather driving conditions.

Logistics is one of the most important elements of a mobile service. For smooth functioning the mobile sonographer requires the help of a competent coordinator to log scheduling calls, to chart sonographer assignments, and to handle calls from the field.

Free-Lancing

Because medical sonography is so technically demanding, a skilled sonographer often is recruited to perform after-hours scanning in private practices or to operate full-time as an independent agent. In some instances the sonographer also must provide the ultrasound instrument and arrange for its transportation and upkeep. Malpractice and liability insurance coverage are highly recommended.

The free-lance sonographer shares many of the same obligations and benefits of the mobile sonographer. In addition to being well-trained, extremely experienced, and independent, he or she also must possess an entrepreneurial spirit and good business and public relations skills.

SUMMARY

Although the hospital is the most complex of the health care organizations, it also provides the broadest benefits. The opportunity to work with both in-patients and out-patients, the opportunity to interact with the multiple subdivisions of medical care, and the opportunity to be involved in teaching or research activities, or both, are incomparable. However, other strong career desires, such as autonomy or specialization, may motivate some sonographers to select employment in one of the alternative areas.

Regardless of the setting the sonographer chooses, there is one common denominator—quality patient care. There also is one common mechanism necessary to reach that goal—teamwork. Even the free-lance sonographer must be a team player. As sonographers we are members of one of the most popular occupations—health care. We need to recognize the valuable contributions of each fellow team member and to work cooperatively with all of them to achieve our mission.

REFERENCES

Craig, M.: The ultrasound suite. Journal of Diagnostic Medical Sonography 1985;1:227-229.

Sternlight, B.: Laboratory development and professional interactions. In Craig, M., editor: Diagnostic Medical Sonography. A Guide to Clinical Practice. Vol. 2: Echocardiography. Philadelphia: J. B. Lippincott Co., 1991.

▼

U N I T   8

Bridging the Gap Between Student and Graduate

LEARNING OBJECTIVES

Students who successfully complete this unit will be able to:

- Describe the attitudinal qualities expected of a diagnostic medical sonographer.

- Describe the functional skills expected of a diagnostic medical sonographer.

- Discuss the need for continuing education and the role played by the American Registry of Diagnostic Medical Sonographers.

- Name at least five sonographic specialties.

- Describe the operational, interpretive, and administrative duties, as well as the ongoing activities of a staff sonographer.

- Compare and contrast the roles of chief sonographer and department manager.

- List and describe at least four nonhospital careers.

Once you overcome the obvious educational and training hurdles that face all student sonographers, you will become aware of other equally important facets of being a good sonographer: those that are more attitudinal than tangible — acquired only through patience and experience. The goal of this unit is to instill an understanding of what is expected of you and the confidence to take you from the familiar, protected world of the student into your professional career.

ATTITUDINAL QUALITIES

Think for a minute of your sonography instructors and the clinical sonographers who have assisted you in your goal of becoming a sonographer. Beyond the memory of their technical abilities, what desirable personal qualities come to mind? As you learn what will be expected of you after graduation, you should be able to match these early role models with the qualities and abilities you hope to acquire and perfect — qualities such as integrity, accountability, and an obvious concern for maintaining high professional standards. Like your early role models, you too will be expected to uphold and promote quality education, to protect and enhance the professional status of sonographers, and to demonstrate leadership to further wider recognition of sonographers within the medical profession and among the general public.

Emotional maturity is expected of graduate sonographers. This quality may be revealed through the use of initiative and independent judgment whenever necessary while always remaining within departmental guidelines, whether working with or without supervision. Acting in a diligent and responsible manner, recognizing and respecting the boundaries of professional closeness to patients, and demonstrating discretion as well as empathy and understanding with regard to patients also are expressions of maturity.

Patience and tenacity are two very important attributes that will help you to see each patient examination to full completion. Recognizing the need to expand some studies to other anatomic areas also is important in your quest to answer the clinical questions.

Most students eagerly await the day when they can put aside their textbooks and actually do the things they have studied and worked so hard to perfect. As you enter the sonography work environment, however, you will become acutely aware of how much more you need to know. You will need motivation to advance beyond your basic skills.

Graduates are expected to maintain competency and to engage in continuing education to remain current with advances in the field. Toward that end, most sonographers seek certification by the American Registry of Diagnostic Medical Sonographers. Although this certificate is voluntary, it is the only currently available means of assuring the medical and lay communities that a sonographer is competent to perform quality diagnostic examinations. Keep in mind, however, that simply acquiring ARDMS certification does not mean that all of your goals have been satisfied.

In addition to developing technical skills, you should bring imagination and artistry to your scanning activities. Each examination should become a personal challenge as you question and confront your fund of knowledge. Graduate sonographers must develop interpersonal skills and a willingness to involve others in their growth. Above all else, they must be *team players* and not soloists!

FUNCTIONAL SKILLS

Full-fledged sonographers should come into the profession with a high degree of technical ability and in-depth knowledge of anatomy and physiology, as well as the basic aspects of clinical medicine. Obviously, knowledge of ultrasound scanning protocols should be thorough. The number of procedures you know depends on your background, training, and particular interests.

Although some sonographers decide to focus on a single specialty, many choose positions that require skill in each of the major sonography specialties. These *general* sonographers should have current knowledge of neurologic, cardiac, vascular, abdominal, obstetric, and gynecologic applications. Like their *specialist* counterparts, they must be capable of dealing effectively with patients and acting quickly in an emergency.

Both groups must have a complete understanding of the complex instrumentation required to ensure its high-quality performance. They also must be capable of deviating from normal techniques whenever necessary, as well as resourceful enough to develop new and better techniques to keep their departments up-to-date.

Sonography students have only a limited opportunity to establish and maintain effective working relationships with patients, employees, physicians, and the general public. The realities of constantly changing and short clinical rotations shield students from the experience of carrying those relationships over longer periods of time — or to conclusion. Some graduates will find themselves thrust into situations in which they must supervise the work activities of back-up sonographers and ancillary personnel.

As a graduate sonographer you will be expected to complete more patient examinations than you did as a student. In whatever work situation you find yourself, you must learn to organize your work so well that you are able to provide each patient with a quality examination that is complete and that facilitates diagnosis. Expertise will develop with experience, but in the beginning, do not hesitate to ask for and follow the advice of your supervisor and co-workers. The following are several commonsense guides for a new graduate to remember:

- *Ask* . . . whenever in doubt about a scanning procedure or patient care technique.
- *Know* . . . when and to whom to report significant patient symptoms.
- *Acquaint yourself* . . . with your department and how it functions: hours, duties, supplies, resources, and intradepartmental as well as interdepartmental conduct.
- *Become knowledgeable* . . . about your institution's emergency, fire, and disaster regulations and procedures.

Your interpretive decisions will play a crucial role in patient diagnosis; therefore you must possess the writing and verbal skills necessary to communicate effectively with physicians, other health care workers, and patients.

Full-time sonographers often are required to work shifts or in an on-call capacity. This may mean working with less supervision and working at times when the usual staff or institutional resources are not available. Although you will be more "on your own" in these instances, again, you should not hesitate to seek assistance whenever you have questions.

In time, you may wish to develop additional skills in specialties such as vascular, neurologic, and high-resolution sonography. For each specialty area you wish to master, you must have a broad appreciation of the anatomy, physiology, pathophysiology, and imaging skills particular to that area. Once sufficient clinical experience has been achieved, you should take on the challenge of passing the registry examinations governing that specialty.

HOSPITAL-BASED CAREER OPPORTUNITIES

Staff Sonographer

In large departments staff sonographers usually are classified by their level of experience. Novice staff sonographers are expected to perform the most basic functions, whereas more experienced sonographers will be given more responsibility and autonomy.

Operations

The following list describes the operational duties expected of hospital-based sonographers.

1. Check requisitions for completeness and procedure requested; refer any questions to the supervising sonologist before beginning the sonography procedure.
2. Review the patient's chart to obtain pertinent clinical history; correlate laboratory data and other diagnostic test results. If necessary, consult with referring physicians regarding a patient's medical history and/or the clinical questions that prompted the sonography request.
3. Position patients correctly for the requested examination; explain the procedure to the patient and give necessary instructions for its completion.
4. Perform emergency examinations (either in the department or at the bedside) with physician supervision.

Instrumentation

The sonographer has the following responsibilities:

1. To knowledgeably operate all necessary diagnostic ultrasound equipment (A-mode, M-mode, B-mode, real-time, and Doppler techniques)
2. To select appropriate transducers (e.g., choosing type, frequency, diameter) for performance of the examination
3. To use ancillary devices (e.g., oscilloscopes, cameras, recorders, strip-charts) to permanently record the diagnostic images
4. To conduct quality-control checks of ultrasound and recording equipment and to record results in an equipment log; to calibrate ultrasound and recording equipment as needed

Interpretation

The sonographer has the following responsibilities:

1. To recognize the significance of all visualized structures and to be able to differentiate artifacts from anatomic or pathologic structures. If any equipment limitations are encountered, apprise the supervising sonologist of the situation.
2. To recognize a diagnostic scan and appreciate the possible need to expand the scope of the study to include other anatomic areas and/or the use of other sonographic techniques.
3. With proper authorization, to render the supervising sonologist's

initial interpretations to the referring physician if a "stat" report is required.

Administration

The hospital-based sonographer has the following duties:

1. To develop and/or maintain a departmental procedure manual
2. To maintain cleanliness of all equipment and of the scanning area; to maintain supplies for the unit or assigned room
3. To fill out all forms (e.g., chronologic log, charge slips) and to create filing materials (film jackets/file folders) for each patient study
4. To record and make copies of teaching- or research-quality examinations
5. To keep records on all equipment, recording service calls and any resulting repairs in an equipment log
6. To establish and maintain good working relationships and rapport with referring physicians, hospital staff, patients, and commercial representatives

Ongoing sonographic responsibilities

The hospital-based sonographer has the following ongoing responsibilities:

1. To evaluate new products and equipment as requested
2. To demonstrate or teach sonographic techniques and clinical applications to students, visiting sonographers, nurses, interns, residents, fellows, and physicians
3. To provide impromptu demonstrations and/or explanations to patients, family, visitors
4. To review pathology, surgery, and delivery reports concerning previously scanned patients for follow up; to use these data to evaluate the accuracy of the sonography studies performed in your facility
5. To maintain currency by reading journals and attending local study groups, annual conventions, seminars, and symposia
6. To contribute to departmental and/or institutional in-service education programs

Chief Sonographer

In addition to performing all of the tasks of the staff sonographer, the chief sonographer should be able to do the following:

1. Work without supervision but within guidelines established in the departmental policies and procedures manual.
2. Gain knowledge of all department equipment, accessories, and operating procedures; develop the ability to diagnose basic equipment malfunctions and communicate them to service personnel.
3. Maintain records of revenues and expenditures and so on; review monthly budgets for accuracy and report any discrepancies.
4. Secure supplies for the sonography section.
5. Recognize and recommend action (as necessary) for improvement of department functions.
6. Coordinate activities of staff sonographers; mediate problems regarding staffing, scheduling, salary reviews and adjustments, discipline, morale, and so on. Provide input as requested on hiring, promoting, or terminating employees.
7. Take responsibility for patient flow and patient care within the sonography department.
8. Conduct inspections of the facility to ensure patient and sonographer safety.

Department Manager

Ideally, the manager of a sonography department should be a sonographer with management training or experience. A combination of skills is important, because this individual must serve as the conduit (and sometimes the buffer) among administration, physicians, sonographers and other employees, and patients.

Courses such as health care administration, management principles, introduction to data processing, statistics, industrial relations or personnel management, financial accounting, health care administration, health planning, and the legal aspects of health services administration are offered at many colleges and universities. If local institutions do not offer degrees in health administration, a course in business administration should be considered (accounting, economics, finance, law, management, marketing, and personnel management and labor relations).

Some of the major responsibilities of a department manager are as follows:

1. Supervising (a) the professional and support staff and (b) the scheduling activities of the department (patients and staff)
2. Assuming responsibility for the communication and practice of departmental and institutional policies, procedures, regulations, and information

3. Handling personnel affairs (evaluations, promotions, raises) and union negotiations
4. Preparing or assisting in developing a budget, controlling inventory, and coordinating departmental purchasing (final decisions and authorizations)
5. Overseeing quality assurance testing
6. Participating in decision making and planning of the immediate, intermediate, and long-term goals of the department.

NONHOSPITAL CAREERS

Unit 7 describes various nonhospital settings in which sonographers perform patient examinations. In this unit we continue exploring career opportunities that are not primarily hospital-based or directly related to patient services.

Teaching

With the dynamic growth and acceptance of diagnostic ultrasound and sonography techniques came the critical need for educators skilled in sonography. Initial "teaching" occurred informally in a show-and-tell fashion. Over time, sonographers (the individuals usually drafted to perform early teaching chores) realized that they would need additional formal training in teaching techniques. As the demands for sonography services increased, they also produced a corresponding demand for the development of educational and training programs inside and *outside* the hospital environment.

Sonography instructors may be active in didactic or clinical settings, or both. One of their primary duties is to develop a course curriculum and operational plans. Classroom instructional techniques may be gained through educational degree programs at the college or university level, as well as from seminars, symposia, and textbooks.

Sonographer-educators also are called on to supervise and evaluate student progress, to maintain student records, to schedule student assignments, and to counsel students in both didactic and clinical settings.

The rewards of teaching are immeasurable, but to be effective, candidates for this profession also must possess a love of working with students and the highest professional standards befitting a role model.

Research

Sonographers who thrive on intellectual stimulation and who are not content until they discover the "whys and wherefores" possess the basic traits of a researcher. Along with the excitement of discovery, however, goes the task of performing detailed investigations and recording large amounts of data.

Research positions exist within universities, hospitals, or commercial manufacturing facilities. Sonography experience and a strong science background are important assets, and, in addition, some positions may require an advanced science degree.

Communication skills, both verbal and written, are essential, as are precision and tenacity.

Commercial

The most common entryway into the field of commercial ultrasound is as an applications specialist. This position involves providing customer training and support, as well as a great deal of travel.

Applications specialists must possess an excellent grasp of the physical principles of diagnostic ultrasound and of all types of ultrasound instrumentation manufactured by their employers. They must be prepared to perform didactic and clinical demonstrations, to conduct patient examinations, to consult with physicians regarding interpretation, to plan and implement customer courses, and to represent their company as exhibitors at medical meetings. Their opinions and evaluations also will be sought by research and development colleagues, and they may be expected to write procedures manuals, to develop teaching slides and tapes, and to contribute to advertising brochures.

The nature of their job requires them to work without direct supervision most of the time and therefore demands an extensive knowledge of sonographic technique and interpretation, pertinent clinical medicine, equipment operation and basic repairs, and professional conduct.

The second most common commercial career opportunity is in ultrasound equipment sales. Once again, the sonographer-salesperson must possess all the requisite skills of a sonographer and also have—or be willing to develop—sales skills and an understanding of business and finance. Extensive travel is required, along with the ability to coordinate both the shipping and installation of equipment and the services of applications specialists and service engineers.

Sales representatives are expected to interact with engineers, other salespersons, and each of the major functionaries in a commercial ultrasound setting (such as advertising, education, finance). They also are required to deal directly with physicians, department managers, sonographers, and purchasing agents. Like the applications specialists, salespersons will be required to handle company exhibits at medical conventions and shows. Because of their wide exposure to both the commercial and scientific areas of medical sonography, they should be willing to serve as resources of information. As a result they must continuously strive to keep abreast of all aspects of the field.

Communications

The need for disseminating diagnostic medical ultrasound information has steadily increased. The communications aspects of medical sonography include a variety of endeavors such as writing, lecturing, and audiovisual production.

Communications skills, orientation to details, ability to write and speak effectively, and to meet deadlines are only a few important attributes. Sonographers who also possess experience or degrees in journalism, public speaking, photography, art, or film production are the strongest candidates for such positions.

Law

The steady rise in ultrasound-related lawsuits has focused attention on the need for attorneys with knowledge of sonography. A small number of sonographers have entered law school with the goal of becoming advocates for sonography personnel or patients, or both. It is still too early to define the complete dimensions or requirements of this developing career opportunity, but it undoubtedly will present an interesting career option.

SUMMARY

The roles and functions of a sonographer are multiple, varied, and still evolving. At first glance performing sonography examinations appears deceptively simple because the basic operational concept is not difficult to understand. On closer inspection, it becomes apparent that the person wielding the ultrasound transducer will have a profound effect on the quality of the examination and will require in-depth education and training if the greatest possible diagnostic benefits are to be realized.

The prerequisites for a sonographer candidate are many. They include intellectual curiosity, emotional maturity, the ability to conceptualize images in three dimensions, paramedical background, demonstrated psychomotor skills, and the ability to interact skillfully with people (physicians, patients, and other health care professionals).

Sonographers perform sonographic studies of patients to gather diagnostic data. Although such studies may be performed in a variety of settings, they should always be carried out under the direct or indirect supervision and responsibility of a qualified physician.

The independent judgment of sonographers is critical because of the need to tailor sonographic examinations to each particular patient's disease process and body habitus. This judgment can be refined only by the sonographer's knowledge of anatomy, physiology, pathophysiology, and relevant clinical medicine and laboratory findings. Differential diagnosis also is an integral part of any sonography study in which pathologic conditions are found, and it is in this regard that sonographers often have been compared to physician assistants.

Sonographers must master the intricacies of ultrasound instrumentation if they expect to overcome any scanning difficulties that might arise.

Interpersonal skills are required because sonographers are expected to discuss procedures with sonologists, referring physicians, other health professionals, and patients. Each type of discussion requires a different approach and intent.

Last, the modern sonographer is almost always cast in the role of teacher to students, staff members, and patients. Therefore, as members of an evolving specialty and seekers of professional autonomy, sonographers must mold every thought, word, and deed toward maintaining the highest of professional standards.

The field of sonography is many things. It is clinically valuable, exciting, and seemingly limited only by our imaginations. On behalf of all sonographers, past and present, I encourage you to remember that your sonography education is a very valuable and powerful tool that will help you get somewhere in life. Once you are "there," however, it is *you* who must make the most of every day.

APPENDIX 1

Common Medical Abbreviations

As you begin the clinical rotation phase of your sonography training, you will be expected to review patients' charts in order to correlate relevant clinical data. This information, along with the sonographic images recorded during the examination, will be used to reach a sonographic diagnosis.

To streamline and expedite the reading and writing of chart data, common medical abbreviations have evolved. The following list contains terms that appear frequently on requisitions, charts, and reports. Although this is by no means a complete listing of medical abbreviations, it represents those a sonographer needs to know.

aa	Of each
AAA	Abdominal aortic aneurysm
Ab	Abortion
ac	before meals
AFM	After fatty meal
AFP	Alpha-fetoprotein
ALL	Acute leukocytic leukemia
AML	Acute monocytic leukemia
Amnio	Amniocentesis
A-mode	Amplitude modulation
AODM	Adult onset of diabetes mellitus
AP	Abdominal perimeter, *or* anteroposterior
ASAP	As soon as possible
ATN	Acute tubular necrosis

BD	Binocular distance
BE	Barium enema
B-H	Braxton Hicks contraction
bid	twice a day
B-mode	Brightness modulation
BMR	Basal metabolism rate
BMT	Bone marrow transplantation
BP	Blood pressure
BPD	Biparietal diameter
BPH	Benign prostatic hypertrophy
BPM	Beats per minute
BPP	Biophysical profile
BSO	Bilateral salpingo-oophorectomy
BTD	Biliary tract disease
BUN	Blood urea nitrogen
Bx	Biopsy
C	Celsius (centrigrade)
c	with
CBC	Complete blood cell count
CBD	Common bile duct
cc	cubic centimeter
CHD	Common hepatic duct
CHF	Congestive heart failure
CI	Cephalic index
CL	Corpus luteum
cm	centimeter
CML	Chronic myeloid leukemia
CNS	Central nervous system
c/o	complains of
Cr	Creatinine
CRL	Crown-rump length
CRT	Cathode-ray tube
CS	Cesarean section
CSF	Cerebrospinal fluid
CST	Contraction stress test
CT	Computed tomography
CVA	Cerebrovascular accident
CVS	Chorionic villus sampling
Cx	Cervix
db	decibel
D&C	Dilatation and curettage
DGC	Depth-gain compensation
dr	dram
DTR	Deep tendon reflex

DT's	Delirium tremens
Dx	Diagnosis
ECG	Echocardiogram
EDC	Estimated date of confinement
EEG	Electroencephalogram, *or* echoencephalogram
EFW	Estimated fetal weight
EKG (ECG)	Electrocardiogram
ETOH	Ethanol (alcohol)
EUA	Examination under anesthesia
F	Fahrenheit
FDIU	Fetal death in utero
FH	Fundal height, *or* fetal heart, *or* family history
FHT	Fetal heart tones
FSH	Follicle-stimulating hormone
F/U	Follow-up
FUO	Fever of unknown origin
FTT	Failure to thrive
Fx	Function
G	Gravida
GA	Gestational age
GB	Gallbladder
GI	Gastrointestinal
gm, g	gram
gr	grain
GS	Gestational sac
GTD	Gestational trophoblastic disease
gtt	drops
GU	Genitourinary
Gyn	Gynecology
HBP	High blood pressure
HC	Head circumference, *or* hepatocellular
HCG	Human chorionic gonadotropin
HCT	Hematocrit
Hg	Mercury
Hgb, Hg	Hemoglobin
HLA	Human leukocyte antigen
HMG	Human menopausal gonadotropin
HP	Head perimeter
hs	at bedtime
HSM	Hepatosplenomegaly
Hx	History
Hydro	Hydrocephalus, *or* hydronephrosis

IC	Iliac crest
IDDM	Insulin-dependent diabetes mellitus
IM	Intramuscular
IPPB	Intermittent positive pressure breathing
IUCD (IUD)	Intrauterine contraceptive device
IUFD (IUD)	Intrauterine fetal demise
IUGR	Intrauterine growth retardation
IUP	Intrauterine pregnancy
IV	Intravenous
IVC	Inferior vena cava
IVP	Intravenous pyelogram
IVS	Interventricular septum
JODM	Juvenile-onset diabetes mellitus
K	Potassium
Kg	kilogram
LCM	Left costal margin
LE	Lower extremity
LFT	Liver function tests (e.g., SGPT [ALT]; SGOT [AST])
LH	Luteinizing hormone
LIF	Long internal focus (transducer)
LK	Left kidney
LLQ	Left lower quadrant
LMP	Last menstrual period
LNMP	Last normal menstrual period
LPO	Left posterior oblique
LSO	Left salpingo-oophorectomy
LSU	Left side up
LT	Ligamentum teres
Lt	Left
LUQ	Left upper quadrant
LV/HW	Lateral-ventricle/hemispheric width ratio
mEq	milliequivalent
mg	milligram
MHz	Megahertz
MI	Myocardial infarction
MIF	Medium internal focus (transducer)
mIU	milli-International unit
ML	Midline
ml	milliliter
mm	millimeter
M-mode, TM	Motion modulation, *or* time-motion modulation
MRI	Magnetic resonance imaging

NGT	Nasogastric tube
NMR	Nuclear magnetic resonance (see *MRI*)
NPO	Nothing by mouth
NSS	Normal size and shape
NST	Nonstress test
NSVD	Normal spontaneous vaginal delivery
NTD	Neural tube defect
OA/OP	Occiput anterior/occiput posterior
Ob	Obstetrics
OC	Ocular diameter
OCG	Oral cholecystogram
OCT	Oxytocin challenge test
OFD	Occipital-frontal diameter
OR	Operating room
oz	ounce
P	after
PA	Popliteal artery, *or* popliteal aneurysm
Para	Number of full-term pregnancies, *or* premature births, *or* abortions, *or* living children
pc	after meals
PE	Pleural effusion, *or* pulmonary embolus
PID	Pelvic inflammatory disease
POC	Products of conception
POD #	Postop day (# _____)
Postop	After surgery
PP	Postpartum
PPD	Test for tuberculosis
prn	as needed
PROM	Premature rupture of membranes
Preop	Before surgery
PSI	Postsaline injection
PT	Pregnancy test
pt	patient
PTA	Prior to admission
PTT	Prothrombin time
PV	Portal vein
qd	every day
qh	every hour
qid	four times a day
qs	sufficient quantity
RBC	Red blood cell
RCM	Right costal margin

Rh	Rhesus
RK	Right kidney
RLL	Right lower lobe
RLQ	Right lower quadrant
R/O	Rule out
RPO	Right posterior oblique
RSO	Right salpingo-oophorectomy
RT	Real-time (dynamic imaging)
RUQ	Right upper quadrant
Rx	Treatment
s	without
SBE	Subacute bacterial endocarditis
SD	Standard deviation
SIF	Short internal focus (transducer)
SMA	Superior mesenteric artery
SMV	Superior mesenteric vein
SP	Splenic vein, *or* symphysis pubis
S/P	Status post
sp gr	specific gravity
stat	immediately
SVD	Spontaneous vaginal delivery
TAB	Therapeutic abortion
TAH	Total abdominal hysterectomy
TAS	Transabdominal scan
TCG, TGC	Time-compensated gain, time-gain compensation
TIA	Transient ischemic attack
tid	three times a day
TIUV	Total intrauterine volume
tko	to keep open (re: intravenous line)
TOA	Tubo-ovarian abscess
Tr	Transverse
TURP	Transurethral resection of the prostate
TVH	Total vaginal hysterectomy
TVS	Transvaginal scan
Tx	Transplant, *or* transducer
U	Umbilicus
UE	Upper extremity
UGI	Upper gastrointestinal series
UPJ	Ureteropelvic junction
URI	Upper respiratory tract infection
U/S	Ultrasound

UTI	Urinary tract infection
UVJ	Ureterovesical junction
VTX	Vertex presentation
WBC	White blood cell
XP	Xyphoid process

A P P E N D I X   2

Medical Terminology

To master medical terminology it is helpful to learn the root words and the prefixes and suffixes that commonly are incorporated into medical terms. The source or origin of a word is called a *root word*.

ROOT WORDS

Angi(o)-	vessel
arth(o)-	joint
cardi(o)-	heart
cephal(o)-	head
cerebr(o)-	brain
chole-, chol(o)-	bile
chondri(o)-	cartilage
cost(o)-	rib
crani(o)-	skull
cyst(o)-	bladder
encephal(o)-	brain
enter(o)-	intestine
gastr(o)-	stomach
hem(o)-, hem(a)-	blood
hepat(o)-	liver
hyster(o)-	uterus
leuk(o)-, leuc(o)-	white
lith(o)-	stone
nephr(o)-	kidney

oste(o)-	bone
phren(o)-	diaphragm
pneum(o)-	air
pyel(o)-	pelvis
viscer(o)-	organ

PREFIXES

a-, an-	absent or deficient
ab-	away from
adeno-	glandular
an-	absent or deficient
ante-	front
anti-	against
arthro-	pertaining to joints
bi-	two
brachio-	arm
cardio-	heart
co-	together
colo-	colon or large intestine
contra-	against
cysto-	bladder
dactyl-	pertaining to fingers or toes
decub-	side
dors-	back
dys-	difficult or painful
ecto-	outside
encephalo-	pertaining to brain
endo-	within
entero-	pertaining to the intestines
epi-	upon
gastro-	pertaining to the stomach
hema-, hemo-	pertaining to blood
hemi-	half
hepato-	pertaining to liver
hydro-	pertaining to water
hyper-	above; a greater concentration
hypo-	below; a lesser concentration
ileo-	refers to small intestine or ileum
infero-	below
inter-	between
intra-	within
lipo-	fat
mal-	disorder
megalo-	large
meningo-	pertaining to membranes surrounding the brain

meno-	pertaining to menstruation
meta-	after or changing
myelo-	spinal cord
myo-	muscle
nephro-	pertaining to the kidney
neuro-	pertaining to nerve or nerves
olig-, oligo-	too little or too few
oro-	pertaining to the mouth
osteo-	pertaining to bone
pan-	all
para-	beside or beyond
peri-	around
phlebo-	pertaining to vein or veins
pneumo-	pertaining to air, lung, breathing
poly-	many, too much
post-	back, after
pre-	before
psycho-	mental
pulmo-	lung
pyelo-	pelvis (renal)
pyo-	pus
retro-	backward
sclero-	hard
sub-	under/below
super-	over/above
trans-	across
vent-	front

SUFFIXES

-algia	pain
-centesis	puncture
-dia	through
-dynia	pain
-ectasis	expansion
-ectomy	surgical removal
-emia	a condition of the blood
-genic	origin
-glycemia	pertaining to blood sugar levels
-iasis	condition
-itis	inflammation
-oid	like
-oma	tumor
-osis	abnormal condition or process
-pathy	abnormality
-phobia	abnormal fear

-plasty	surgical correction
-ptosis	falling or drooping
-rhaphy	suture
-scopy	inspection
-tomy	incision
-uria	contained within the urine

A P P E N D I X   3

Glossary

The following list contains medical and technical words that are often used on patient charts and in sonography textbooks. This is by no means a complete listing of what a sonographer needs to know. For further study you may wish to check any one of the many excellent medical dictionaries available in the hospital library.

A

abdomen: The large inferior cavity of the trunk, extending from the diaphragm to the brim of the pelvis. It is artificially divided into nine regions: right hypochondriac; epigastric; left hypochondriac; right lumbar; umbilical; left lumbar; right inguinal; hypogastric; left inguinal. **acute a.,** an acute pathologic condition within the belly, which requires prompt surgical intervention.

abduction: Withdrawal of a part from the axis of the trunk or an extremity.

aberrant: Varying/deviating from normal form, structure, or course.

abortion: The expulsion of the embryo or fetus from the uterus any time before week 28 of pregnancy, either by natural or by artificially induced means. When this occurs during the first 3 months, it is termed *abortion;* from this time to viability, *miscarriage;* and from the period of viability to full term, *premature delivery/birth.* Types of abortions are **artificial a.,** intentional premature termination of pregnancy by medicinal/mechanical means. **complete a.,** the total expulsion of all products of conception from the uterus. **criminal a.,** illegal interference with progress of pregnancy, or *illegal abortion.* **habitual a.,** accidental abortion recurring in successive pregnancies. **incomplete a.,** partial expulsion of the products of conception. **inevitable a.,** an abortion that has advanced to a stage in which termination of pregnancy can no longer be prevented. **missed a.,** a condition in which the fetus has died but the products of conception are not expelled within 2 weeks. **partial a.,** premature expulsion of one fetus in the presence of multiple gestation. **spontaneous a.,** unexpected premature expulsion of the products of conception when no abortive agents have been applied. **therapeutic a.,** termination of a pregnancy that poses a hazard to the life of the mother. **threatened a.,** occurrence of signs/symptoms of impending loss of the embryo/fetus. May be prevented by treatment or may go on to inevitable abortion. **tubal a.,** escape of the products of conception through the abdominal opening of the fallopian tube into the peritoneal cavity.

abruptio: A tearing away. **a. placentae,** premature separation of the placenta.

abscess: A pus-filled cavity that can develop anywhere, for example, on the skin or in any internal organ. Antibiotics may be helpful, but draining may be necessary to remove the pus.

acute: Describes sudden onset of relatively severe or sharp manifestations that run a short course. Acute problems may be mild or severe.

Addison's disease: A disease resulting from decreased function of the adrenal glands.

adduction: Any movement of one part or a limb toward another or toward the midline of the body.

adhesion: Abnormal union of an organ or part to another. **fibrous a.,** firm attachment of adjacent serous membranes by bands or masses of fibrous connective tissue; caused by organization and scarring of exudates, resulting from infection or partial destruction of the surfaces.

adipose: Fatty, fatlike.

adnexa: Accessory parts or appendages of an organ.

adrenaline: Also known as *epinephrine.* A hormone produced by the adrenal glands. Available in drug form to improve breathing for persons with asthma, to treat severe allergic reactions, or to stimulate the heart in cardiac arrest.

airway: A respiratory passage. Any of several devices used to maintain a clear and unobstructed respiratory passage.

albuminuria: Presence of protein or albumin in the urine.

ambulatory: Walking or able to walk; designating a patient not confined to bed.

amenorrhea: Absence of menses.

amniography: Radiographic visualization of the fetus by injection of a dye through the abdominal wall and into the amniotic sac.

analgesia: The absence of pain; usually denotes relief of pain without loss of consciousness.

anasarca: Massive generalized edema.

anastamosis: The joining together of structures.

anemia: Low level of hemoglobin, the red blood cell chemical that carries oxygen to body tissues.

aneurysm: Weakening of a blood vessel because of disease, age, injury, or congenital defect. Rupture of the weakened wall is usually life-threatening.

angina: Severe, often choking chest pain.

angiogram: Visualization of the blood vessels with x-ray examination.

angioplasty: Surgical opening of a clogged blood vessel by inflating a balloon and stretching the wall. Often performed after heart attack, along with the administration of clot-dissolving medication.

anoxia: Lack of oxygen; absence of oxygen in the tissues.

antibody: An immunoglobulin molecule that reacts specifically with a substance (antigen) that induced its synthesis or with a closely related antigen.

antigen: Any substance that induces the formation of antibodies with which it reacts specifically.

antiseptic: An agent that inhibits microorganisms.

anuria: Lack of urine production; absence of excretion of urine from the body.

aorta: The main artery through which blood leaves the heart for distribution to the rest of the body.

aphasia: Defect or loss of power of expression in speech, writing, or signs or loss of comprehension of spoken or written language because of injury or disease of brain centers.

aplasia: Lack of development of an organ or tissue or of the cellular products from an organ or tissue.

apnea: Cessation of breathing for short periods of time (sleep apnea) or for prolonged and potentially life-threatening times (e.g., in premature babies).

arrhythmia: Abnormality of heart rate or rhythm, or both.

arteriosclerosis: Hardening and loss of elasticity of the arterial wall. Common with aging and in certain diseases. Term often used interchangeably with *atherosclerosis,* a thickening of the inner wall of blood vessels from cholesterol deposits.

ascites: An abnormal collection of serous fluid in the peritoneal cavity.

aseptic: Sterile, free of microorganisms.

asymptomatic: Showing or causing no symptoms.

ataxia: Failure of muscular coordination.

atherosclerosis: A form of arteriosclerosis.

atrophy: Diminution in the size of a cell, tissue, or organ.

autoclave: A device that sterilizes by steam under pressure.

autonomic nervous system: Part of the nervous system that regulates involuntary life-maintaining activities such as heart beat, respiration, and hormone secretion.

azotemia: An excess of urea or other nitrogenous substances in the blood.

B

bacteria: Microbes or organisms, some of which cause disease and some of which live peacefully within the body, aiding such functions as digestion.

benign: Harmless; nonmalignant character of a neoplasm.

bilateral: Affecting both sides.

biopsy: Removal of a small sample of tissue for microscopic examination.

brachial: Region between the elbow and shoulder.

bradycardia: Abnormally slow pulse.

bronchi: Major air passageways in the lungs.

bronchoscopy: Direct examination of the bronchus.

C

calculus: A stonelike formation, usually composed of mineral salts.

cannula: A small tube for insertion into a body cavity.

carcinogen: An environmental agent that can produce cancer.

carcinoma: Malignant neoplasm arising from certain tissues. *Carcinoma in situ* describes an early stage of cancer that is highly curable because it has not spread (metastasized) beyond its origin; cancer.

cardiology: Medical specialty that deals with disorders of the heart and cardiac vesculature.

catheterize: The introduction of a hollow tube into a body cavity, such as the urinary bladder, to draw off fluid.

cerebral vascular accident (CVA): Pathologic condition of a blood vessel in the brain—either rupture or occlusion, with formation of a blood clot.

chemotherapy: Treatment of a disease by means of administering chemicals.

cholecystectomy: Surgical removal of the gallbladder.

cholecystitis: Infection of the gallbladder.

cholecystogram: An x-ray procedure used to visualize the gallbladder.

cholelithiasis: Gallstones.

chronic: Persisting over a long period of time; denoting a disease of slow progress and long continuance.

cirrhosis: Hardening of an organ.

colostomy: Surgical procedure to form an artificial opening into the large bowel.

congenital: Present at birth. Congenital problems can be inherited, the result of infection or drug use in the mother, or the effect of uterine abnormalities.

convulsion: Violent, uncoordinated, involuntary contractions of the muscles.

coronal: A plane parallel to the long axis of the body.

cranial: Referring to the skull.

culdoscopy: Internal visual examination of the female reproductive organs through a small incision in the pouch of Douglas.

cutaneous: Referring to the skin.

cyanosis: Bluish discoloration of the skin and mucous membranes, caused by insufficient oxygen in the blood.

cyst: A sac or cavity filled with fluid or oily material; can form in any part of the body.

cystitis: Inflammation of the urinary bladder.

cystoscopy: Visual examination of the interior of the urinary bladder.

cytology: The study of cells.

D

defecation: Elimination of wastes from the intestine.

diabetes insipidus: A disease caused by a deficiency of antidiuretic hormone (ADH).

diabetes mellitus: A metabolic disease in which carbohydrates are poorly oxidized.

dialysis: Cleansing the blood by artificial means when kidneys have failed. *Hemodialysis* filters blood through a machine; *peritoneal* *dialysis* uses the peritoneal membrane that lines the abdomen to filter impurities.

diaphoresis: Excessive perspiration.

diastole: The relaxation of the heart between contractions.

dilation, dilatation: Enlargement of an opening or a hollow organ or tube.

disinfectant: An agent that kills *some* pathogens.

distal: Farther from the body or from the origin of a part.

diuresis: Increased urine production.

diuretic: A drug used to cause diuresis.

dorsal: The posterior aspect or back of the body or organ.

dorsiflexion: Flexion or bending of the foot toward the leg.

dysfunction: Disturbed or abnormal function of an organ.

dysmenorrhea: Painful menstruation.

dysphagia: Difficulty in swallowing.

dysplasia: Abnormal change or growth; alteration in size, shape, and organization of differentiated cells.

dyspnea: Labored breathing.

dystrophy: Faulty or defective nutrition.

dysuria: Painful or difficult urination.

E

ecchymosis: A bruise; a discoloration of the skin caused by the extravasation of blood.

echocardiogram: Sonographic examination of the heart.

ectopic: Out of place.

edema: Swelling caused by fluid retention; accumulation of abnormally large amounts of fluid in the interstitial spaces.

effusion: Escape of fluid into a space such as the pleural cavity.

elective: Not urgent. Elective surgery can be scheduled at the patient's convenience.

electrocardiogram: A graphic recording of the electrical current produced by the contraction of the heart.

electroencephalogram: A graphic recording of the electrical currents produced by brain action.

electrolyte: A solution, such as a salt solution, that can conduct electricity.

embolus: A mass of undissolved material traveling in the blood; it may be solid, liquid, or gaseous.

embryo: The fetus before the end of the eighth week of conception.

emesis: Vomitus.

emphysema: A chronic lung disease usually characterized by greatly distended alveoli.

empyema: Pus in the pleural cavity.

endogenous: Originating within the body.

endoscope: An instrument used to inspect the interior of a body cavity.

enzyme: A protein that acts as a catalyst in biochemical reactions.

epistaxis: Nosebleed.

erosion: Wearing away of tissue.

erythema: An unusual redness of the skin.

esophagoscopy: Visual examination of the esophagus.

etiology: Study of the cause of a disease or condition.

evisceration: Protrusion of internal organs through a wound.

exacerbation: An increase in the severity or intensity of a disease and any of the symptoms.

excoriation: An area where the skin has been scraped away or chafed.

exogenous: Originating outside of the body.

extension: The increasing or straightening of the angle at a joint.

extrasystole: A premature contraction of the heart; a type of cardiac arrhythmia.

exudate: A substance thrown out, such as pus or serous fluid.

F

fascia: A sheet of fibrous tissue that covers muscles and certain other organs.

feces: Excrement from the bowels.

fetal distress: Abnormal condition of the fetus characterized by irregular heart rhythm and meconium (fetal bowel movement) that discolors amniotic fluid. Turning the mother onto her side and administering oxygen often helps, but early delivery sometimes is necessary.

fetus: The unborn infant.

fibrillation: A type of cardiac arrhythmia.

fibrosis: The formation of fibrous tissue, usually as a reparative process.

filtration: The process by which water and dissolved substances are pushed through a permeable membrane from areas of high pressure to areas of lower pressure.

fissure: A cleft or groove.

fistula: Abnormal channel between two organs or an internal organ and the skin. A deep ulcer or abnormal passage often leading from a hollow organ to the body surface. Sometimes caused by congenital malformation or complications of surgery or childbirth.

flatus: Gas or air in the stomach or intestines.

flexion: Decreasing of the angle at a joint, for example, the bending of the elbow.

fluoroscope: An x-ray machine used to allow visual examination of internal organs and to observe the movement and contour of the organs.

Foley catheter: A tube used for the continuous drainage of urine.

fossa: A shallow or hollow place in a bone.

frontal: A plane that divides the body into front and back portions.

G

gastrectomy: Surgical removal of a part or all of the stomach.

gavage: Feeding by means of a stomach tube.

germicide: An agent that kills germs.

goiter: Enlargement of the thyroid gland.

gynecology: Medical specialty that deals with the reproductive system of the nongravid female.

H

hallucination: Hearing, seeing, or feeling things that do not exist.

heart failure: The inability of the heart muscle to pump blood. Leads to fluid accumulation in the lungs, which makes breathing difficult and causes swelling of the legs, feet, liver, and other internal organs. Also known as *congestive heart failure.*

hematemesis: Bloody vomitus.

hematocrit: The percentage of the volume of a blood sample that contains erythrocytes.

hematology: The study of the blood.

hematoma: A localized mass of extravasated blood as a result of trauma. Usually clotted in an organ, space, or tissue.

hematuria: Blood in the urine.

hemiplegia: Paralysis of one side of the body.

hemodialysis: A procedure to remove waste or other toxic substances from the blood that cannot be eliminated by the kidney.

hemoglobin: Oxygen-carrying substance of the red blood cells.

hemolysis: Destruction of red blood cells.

hemoptysis: Bloody sputum.

hemostasis: Stopping the flow of blood.

hemostat: An instrument or clamp used to stop bleeding.

hernia: Protrusion of an organ or part of an organ through the muscular wall.

hirsutism: Abnormal hairiness.

histology: The study of tissues.

Hodgkin's disease: A malignant disease characterized by swelling of the lymph glands.

homeostasis: The maintenance of constant conditions in the internal environment. Environment of the body tends to return to normal whenever it is disturbed.

hydrotherapy: The use of water in treating disease.

hyperemia: An excess of blood in any part of the body.

hyperglycemia: Excess sugar in the blood.

hyperplasia: An abnormal increase in the number of normal cells in a tissue or organ.

hypertension: A persistently high arterial blood pressure.

hypertrophy: An increase in the size of an organ or part as a result of an increase in the size of its constituent cells.

hypervolemia: An abnormal increase in the circulating blood volume.

hypoplasia: Underdevelopment of tissue or an organ, usually caused by a decrease in the number of cells.

I

iatrogenic: Any adverse condition in a patient that results from treatment by a physician or surgeon (e.g., side effects of medication).

icterus: Jaundice.

idiopathic: Disease or condition whose cause is unknown.

ileostomy: An artificial opening into the ileum.

ileus: Obstruction of the bowel, usually as a result of the inhibition of nerve impulses necessary to the maintenance of normal peristalsis.

incontinence: Inability to hold urine or feces.

induration: Hardening.

infarct: An area of necrosis resulting from a lack of blood supply.

infection: Invasion of the body tissues by microorganisms, with multiplication of the microorganisms in the tissues.

inferior: Lower.

inflammation: A tissue response to injury. The signs are pain, heat, redness, and swelling.

intercostal: Between the ribs.

interstitial: Lying between; the spaces between the cells; intercellular.

intravenous: Within a vein, often meaning an injection into a vein.

invasive: Procedures that involve entering the body; tendency to spread to other parts of the body (e.g., tumors).

involution: The return of an enlarged organ to its normal size.

irradiation: Exposure to any form of radiant energy, such as x-ray or radioisotopes.

ischemia: Decreased blood supply.

J

jaundice: A yellow discoloration of the skin and eyes caused by excessive amounts of bile in the blood. May be normal in newborn infants, but in adults it results from hepatitis, gallstones, or more serious liver problems.

K

ketosis: Disturbance of the acid-base balance of the body.

L

laceration: A wound caused by tearing.

lateral: Toward the side.

lesion: Any pathologic or traumatic change in a tissue.

leukocyte: White blood cell.

ligation: The application of a tie around a vessel or hollow tube, such as the fallopian tubes.

lipoma: Benign collection of fatty tissues.

lithiasis: Stone formation.

lithotomy: Surgical removal of a stone; also a common gynecologic position.

lithotripsy, litholapaxy: Use of sound waves to break up kidney stones or gallstones.

lumbar: Pertaining to the loin.

lumbar puncture: A procedure used to withdraw cerebrospinal fluid.

lymph node: The primary infection fighters.

lymphocyte: A type of white blood cell.

M

malaise: Weakness, lack of energy, and vague sense of bodily discomfort.

malignant: Tending to become progressively worse and to result in death; usually pertains to cancer or other life-threatening conditions.

mammary: Pertaining to the breasts.

mastectomy: The surgical removal of a breast.

menarche: Onset of menstruation.

menopause: The cessation of menstruation at the end of the reproductive period of life.

menorrhagia: Profuse menstrual flow.

menstruation: The periodic discharge of blood and endometrial tissue from the uterus.

metabolism: The chemical processes of life.

metastasis: The transfer of a disease from one part of the body to another.

metrorrhagia: Abnormal bleeding from the uterus during the intermenstrual period.

micturition: The passing of urine.

midsagittal: A plane dividing the body or an organ into right and left halves.

mucous membrane: A type of membrane that lines body cavities that open to the outside of the body.

mucus: A secretion produced by mucous membranes.

multiple sclerosis: A progressive disease of the nervous system.

muscular dystrophy: A progressive disease characterized by wasting of the voluntary muscles.

myasthenia gravis: A disease characterized by progressive paralysis of muscles without any sensory disturbance.

myocardial infarction (MI): Heart attack.

myocardium: The heart muscle.

myoma: A muscle tumor.

myxedema: A disease caused by a deficiency of thyroid hormones.

N

necrosis: The death or decay of one or more cells, or a portion of tissue in which the growth is uncontrolled and progressive; usually results from an interruption of blood supply or injury.

neoplasm: A mass of cells forming a new growth of tissue, such as a tumor, in which the growth is uncontrolled and progressive.

nephrectomy: The surgical removal of a kidney.

nephritis: Inflammation of the kidney.

nephron: A microscopic functional unit in the cortex of the kidney.

nephroptosis: A downward displacement of the kidney.

nephrosis: A kidney disease.

nephrostomy: A surgical procedure involving placement of a tube into the renal pelvis of the kidney for drainage purposes.

neurosis: A psychic or mental illness usually characterized by anxiety and difficulties in adjusting to new or stressful situations.

nocturia: Excessive urination at night.

normal saline: A 0.9% solution of sodium chloride, frequently used for irrigations.

O

obesity: The condition of being excessively overweight.

obstetrics: Medical specialty that deals with pregnancy and childbirth.

occipital: Pertaining to the base of the skull.

occlusion: A blockage.

oliguria: Secretion of a diminished amount of urine.

oophorectomy: The surgical removal of an ovary.

ophthalmoscope: An instrument used to examine the interior of the eye.

organic: Pertaining to living matter.

orifice: The entrance or outlet of a body cavity.

orthopedics: A medical specialty dealing with disorder of the skeletal system.

osseous: Pertaining to bony tissue.

ossification: Bone formation.

osteoarthritis: A chronic degenerative disease of the joints.

osteomyelitis: Infection of the bone.

osteoporosis: A disease in which there is a decrease in bone density.

ovulation: Release of a mature ovum from the ovary.

ovum: The mature female sex cell formed in the ovary.

P

palliative: Treatment that eliminates the symptoms but does not affect the cause of the symptoms.

palpation: Examination of the body by means of feeling with the hand.

palpitation: Rapid heart action felt by the patient.

papillae: Small nipple or finger-shaped elevations.

papule: A small, raised lesion.

paracentesis: The removal of fluid from the peritoneal cavity.

paraplegia: Paralysis of the lower extremities.

parasympathetic: Pertaining to autonomic nerves that originate in the lower part of the brain and the sacral portion of the spinal cord.

parenchyma: The distinguishing or specific cells (functional elements) of a gland or organ as distinct from the connective tissue framework, or stroma.

parietal: Pertaining to the body wall; also the region of the head posterior to the frontal region and anterior to the occipital region.

Parkinson's disease: A progressive disease of the central nervous system characterized by stiffness, slowed movements, and rhythmic, fine tremors of resting muscles.

parturition: The birth of an infant.

pathogen: Anything that causes disease.

pathology: A branch of medicine concerned with structural and functional changes caused by disease.

pectoral: Pertaining to the breast or chest.

pediatrics: A medical specialty that deals with diseases of children.

pelvimetry: Radiographic measurement of the pregnant woman's pelvis to determine whether vaginal delivery is possible.

percussion: A diagnostic procedure in which a part is struck with short, sharp blows to aid in determining the condition of the parts beneath by the sound obtained.

perfusion: A liquid pouring over or through something.

pericardium: The membraneous sac that contains the heart.

perineum: The anatomic region at the lower end of the trunk between the thighs.

peripheral: Away from the center.

peristalsis: Contractions of smooth muscle, causing a wavelike motion.

peritoneum: A serous membrane that surrounds the abdominal organs and lines the abdominal cavity.

peritonitis: Inflammation of the peritoneum.

petechiae: Small hemorrhagic areas.

pH: The symbol relating to the hydrogen ion concentration or activity of a solution to that of a given standard solution.

phenotype: An organism's physical appearance.

phlebitis: Inflammation of veins.

phlebotomy: Insertion of needles into veins.

placebo: A substance that has no pharmacologic action, which is given to satisfy a patient's desire for drug treatment; also used in research to ensure that a medication rather than psychologic factors have caused a response.

placenta: The nutrient and excretory organ of the fetus.

plasma: The fluid portion of the circulating blood.

platelet: One of the formed particles of the blood that is important in clot formation.

pneumonectomy: The surgical removal of a lung.

pneumothorax: Air in the pleural cavity.

polyp: An abnormal growth from a mucous membrane.

polyuria: Greatly increased urinary output.

posterior: Situated behind or toward the rear.

proctoscopy: Visual inspection of the rectum.

prognosis: An opinion of the probable outcome of a disease or injury.

prolapse: Downward displacement of a tissue or organ outside of its normal position.

prophylaxis: The prevention of disease.

prosthesis: An artificial replacement for a part of the body that has been lost.

proximal: Closest to the point of attachment.

pruritus: Itching.

psychogenic: Caused by emotional factors.

psychosis: A severe form of mental illness in which the patient may have hallucinations and personality changes.

psychosomatic: A type of illness in which thought processes may disturb organic functions.

ptosis: A drooping or prolapse of an organ or part.

pulmonary: Pertaining to the lungs.

purulent: Containing pus.

pus: A product of inflammation consisting of fluid, white blood cells, and bacteria.

pustule: A small elevation filled with pus.

pyelonephrosis: Any disease of the kidney and its pelvis.

pyrexia: Fever.

pyuria: Pus in the urine.

Q

quadriplegia: Paralysis of all four extremities.

R

radiation: The emission of radiant energy.

radioactivity: The spontaneous emission of alpha, beta, and/or gamma rays.

radioisotope: A radioactive element used as a tracer in the body because it can be detected and followed by its radioactive emissions.

radiopaque: Not readily penetrated by x-rays.

rale: An abnormal respiratory sound usually associated with fluid in the air passages.

reflux: Backflow of material in the body.

remission: Disappearance of the symptoms of a disease.

renal: Pertaining to the kidney.

resection: Surgical removal of an organ or structure.

resuscitation: Restoration to life or consciousness.

retroperitoneal: Behind the peritoneum.

rheumatoid arthritis: An inflammatory disease of the connective tissue characterized by remissions and exacerbations of pain and stiffness of the joints.

Rh factor: A substance in the red blood cells important in the typing of blood for transfusions and in obstetric care.

rugae: Folds inside some of the hollow organs (e.g., stomach, urinary bladder).

S

sagittal: Pertaining to a plane that divides the body into right and left portions.

salpingitis: Inflammation of the fallopian tubes.

sclerosis: Hardening.

seizure: Convulsion. Sudden, uncontrolled electrical activity in the brain that can cause reactions ranging from mild feelings of fear to loss of consciousness and generalized twitching.

sepsis: Poisoning by bacteria.

septicemia: Bacteria (circulating in the blood) that multiply and produce toxins; blood poisoning.

serosanguineous: Pertaining to or containing both serum and blood.

serum: The fluid portion of the blood obtained after removal of the fibrin clot and blood cells.

sign: An objective manifestation of disease.

spastic: Involuntary muscle spasms.

sperm: The mature male sex cell formed in the testes.

sphincter: A muscle that closes an orifice.

sphygmomanometer: An instrument used to measure blood pressure.

stasis: A stoppage of the flow of any body fluid.

stenosis: Narrowing of a passage.

sterilization: A process by which materials are made free of microorganisms; a procedure that makes an individual incapable of reproduction.

stethoscope: An instrument used to listen to sounds produced within the body.

stricture: A narrowing of a passageway.

subcutaneous: Beneath the skin.

supine: Lying on the back, face upward.

suture: Surgical stitch or the material used to make the stitch.

sympathetic nerves: Fibers of the autonomic nervous system that originate in the thoracic and lumbar regions of the spinal cord.

symphysis pubis: The place where the pubic bones join together; common landmark for pelvic scanning.

symptom: Subjective evidence of disease.

syncope: Fainting.

syndrome: A set of signs and symptoms.

systole: The contraction of the heart.

T

tachycardia: An abnormally fast heart rate. Can be caused by heart problems, fever, an overactive thyroid, or drugs.

temporal: Pertaining to the region of the body anterior to the ear; the temple.

tetany: Muscle twitching and cramps caused by hypocalcemia.

therapy: Treatment.

thoracentesis: A procedure used to remove fluid from the pleural cavity.

thorax: Pertaining to the chest.

thrombosis: Formation of a stationary clot (thrombus) inside a blood vessel.

torsion: Twisting; any organ that moves freely can become twisted. Surgical correction required to deter organ death from lack of blood supply.

toxemia: A general intoxication resulting from the absorption of bacterial products; also may occur in pregnancy for reasons not completely understood.

toxin: A poison.

trauma: Any type of injury.

tremor: Involuntary shaking or trembling.

tumor: Any swelling or new growth.

U

ulcer: An open lesion.

unilateral: Occurring on only one side of the body.

urea: A nitrogenous substance that is one of the end products of protein digestion.

uremia: A condition in which there is an excess accumulation of waste products in the blood stream.

ureter: The tube leading from the kidney to the urinary bladder.

urethra: The tube leading from the urinary bladder to the outside of the body.

urinalysis: Laboratory examination of urine.

urology: A medical specialty that deals with disorders of the urinary system.

V

vaccine: A preparation made from a killed or weakened pathogen.

varices: Enlarged and tortuous veins.

vasodilatation: An increase in blood vessel diameter, particularly the peripheral arterioles.

vasomotor: Presiding over the expansion or contraction of blood vessels.

ventral: Pertaining to the anterior surface.

vertigo: Extreme dizziness.

vesicle: A blister.

viable: Capable of living.

virus: A small disease-causing particle too tiny to be seen by conventional microscopes. Most viral infections are untreatable until the patient's own immune defenses eliminate the virus.

vital capacity: The amount of air that can forcibly be expelled after the largest possible inhalation.

Z

zygote: The fertilized ovum.

APPENDIX 4

Pertinent Clinical Laboratory Tests

An important facet of correlating the patient's physical condition with the diagnostic images obtained during sonographic examination is to review the clinical laboratory tests that have been performed. The selection of basic laboratory tests for this section is not all-inclusive but represents the most commonly encountered tests related to the major imaging specialties of abdominal, cardiac, and obstetric sonography.

Normal values are not expressed because of the variety of standards used in each laboratory.

ENZYME TESTING

Enzymes, which are found in all tissues, are complex compounds that catalyze the biochemical reactions of the body. Each tissue has its own specific enzyme, with one enzyme being common to more than one type of tissue. Enzyme elevation implies that a particular tissue is damaged enough to release significant quantities of the enzyme into the blood (Tilkian and Connover, 1975).

LIVER FUNCTION TESTS

Liver function tests that utilize enzymes are one of the most comprehensive methods to evaluate various physiologic processes.

Serum Glutamic-Oxaloacetic Transaminase

Serum glutamic-oxaloacetic transaminase (SGOT) (AST) is an enzyme present in tissues with a high rate of metabolic activity (e.g., heart muscle, liver, kidney, and red blood cells). After the injury or death of physiologically active cells, SGOT is released into the blood stream. Elevated values will be found 8 hours after injury and should peak in 24 to 36 hours if the original episode is not repeated. Levels usually fall to normal in four to six days. The level of SGOT in the blood is directly proportional to the number of cells damaged and the interval of time between injury and the test.

Serum Glutamic Pyruvate Transaminase

Serum glutamic pyruvate transaminase (SGPT) (ALT) also is liberated from destroyed cells; however, it is more specific than SGOT in evaluating liver function. In the absence of cardiac or other muscle injury, elevations of both SGOT and SGPT are diagnostic of hepatocellular damage.

Mild increases of SGPT are associated with acute cirrhosis, hepatic metastasis, and pancreatitis. Mild to moderate increases are seen in obstructive jaundice. Hepatocellular disease and infectious or toxic hepatitis will produce markedly increased SGPT levels.

Lactic Acid Dehydrogenase

Lactic acid dehydrogenase (LDH) is present in nearly all metabolizing cells, with highest concentrations in tissues of the kidneys, heart, skeletal muscle, brain, liver, and red blood cells. Tissue damage causes this enzyme to be released into the blood stream. Origin of the release cannot be determined by routine examination. Electrophoresis used to separate the isoenzymes of LDH, however, can determine the source of an elevation of this enzyme (Tilkian and Connover, 1975).

Although the LDH test is not specific for hepatic function, in combination with other diagnostic test results, its main use is to indicate the presence of myocardial and pulmonary infarction. Persistent, slightly increased LDH levels are associated with hepatitis, cirrhosis, and obstructive jaundice.

Alkaline Phosphatase

Alkaline phosphatase is an enzyme produced by the liver and bone, as well as by the placenta during pregnancy. In the absence of either bone disease or pregnancy, marked increases of alkaline phosphatase are associated with obstructive jaundice, hepatic carcinoma, abscess, and cirrhosis. Moderate elevations are seen in hepatitis and less active cases of cirrhosis. Extreme elevations in patients with normal liver function suggest the possibility of Paget's disease of the bone along with osteogenic sarcoma or metastatic carcinoma to the bone (Ferguson, 1984).

Bilirubin

Bilirubin is the chief bile pigment in humans. Resulting from the breakdown of hemoglobin in worn-out red blood cells, bilirubin — along with lecithin, cholesterol, and inorganic salts — is secreted as bile by the liver cells. Disruption of this production cycle can occur in three major ways: (1) excessive amounts of red blood cell destruction, (2) malfunction of the liver cells, or (3) blockage of the ducts leading from the cells. When disruptions cause an increased level of serum bilirubin, this bile pigment eventually leaks into the tissues, producing a yellow caste to the skin and the white of the eyes (jaundice).

Total bilirubin is a screening procedure for detecting elevated bilirubin levels. It is a nonspecific test. Two further tests are required to specify the cause of clinical jaundice.

Indirect bilirubin, or unconjugated bilirubin, is protein-bound in the serum. Elevated levels are associated with red blood cell destruction (e.g., hemolytic anemias, trauma in the presence of large hematoma, or hemorrhagic pulmonary infarcts) (Ferguson, 1984).

Direct bilirubin, or conjugated bilirubin, circulates freely in the blood. Upon reaching the liver, it is conjugated with glucuronic acid and is excreted into the bile. Elevations usually are caused by obstructive jaundice. Obstructive (surgical) jaundice generally results from an obstruction of the biliary system caused by the formation of stones or neoplasms.

Specific disease processes that cause an elevation of both direct and indirect bilirubin levels — with marked increases in the direct level — are hepatic metastasis, hepatitis, lymphoma, cholestasis as a result of drug use, and cirrhosis (Ferguson, 1984).

Prothrombin Time and Vitamin K Administration Test

Prothrombin is a liver enzyme that is part of the blood-clotting mechanism. The production of prothrombin depends on adequate intake and utilization of vitamin K.

The increase of prothrombin time in liver disease may be the result of either malabsorption of the fat-soluble vitamin K or a deficiency in the formation of one of the clotting factors. Prolongation of prothrombin time manifests by bleeding tendencies (Tilkian and Connover, 1975). Persistently increased prothrombin time is associated with the presence of severe liver disease, with accompanying cellular damage (e.g., cirrhosis and metastatic disease).

BILIARY SYSTEM

The function of the biliary system is to transport bile, which is produced continuously by the hepatic parenchymal cells, to the duodenum, where it aids in digestion. Bile also is useful in emulsifying and promoting the absorption of fats, as well as in facilitating the actions of lipase, a pancreatic enzyme. After digestion occurs, the bile is released, by the contraction of the gallbladder, into the biliary system and finally into the duodenum.

SGOT and SGPT Levels

SGOT—and more specifically SGPT—values can be mildly to moderately elevated in cases of biliary system obstruction. Such obstruction can cause biliary regurgitation that, if prolonged, can result in hepatic cell damage.

Alkaline Phosphatase

In the presence of biliary disease (e.g., obstructive jaundice) alkaline phosphatase values are *markedly* increased.

Direct/Indirect Bilirubin

Direct bilirubin values are elevated not only in obstructive jaundice but also in hepatic metastasis, hepatitis, and lymphoma. In the latter conditions, however, the indirect bilirubin level also is elevated. The nonspecificity of these laboratory tests often prompts requests for the sonographer to differentiate between medical and surgical causes of the jaundice.

PANCREAS

As both an endocrine and an exocrine gland, the pancreas is an organ with complex functions. Its endocrine functions cause the secretion of hormones (insulin and glucagon), produced by the islets of Langerhans, directly into the blood stream. Insulin provides the major control over carbohydrate metabolism, and glucagon aids in the process.

Sonographers are primarily interested in the exocrine functions of the pancreas: the production of digestive enzymes from pancreatic acinar cells. After release and travel through the acinar ducts, the duct of Wirsung, and the common bile duct, enzymes eventually travel to the duodenum. The digestive enzymes trypsin, lipase, and amylase aid in the digestion of proteins, fats, and starches.

Direct Bilirubin

Various pancreatic pathologic processes cause obstruction of the ampulla of Vater or the common bile duct, or both. Such obstructions are reflected by elevated levels of bilirubin. Conjugated or direct bilirubin levels are associated with carcinoma of the head of the pancreas and acute pancreatitis that produces an obstruction.

Amylase

Amylase, an enzyme produced within the pancreas, as well as in other organs such as the salivary glands and liver, aids in converting starches to sugars.

Increased amylase levels in the blood are associated with inflammation of the pancreas. Elevations greatly increase within 3 to 6 hours after the appearance of clinical symptoms, and levels remain elevated for approximately 24 hours after acute episodes. Other causes of elevated amylase values include chronic pancreatitis (acute attack), partial gastrectomy, obstruction of the pancreatic duct, perforated peptic ulcer, alcoholic poisoning, acute cholecystitis, and intestinal obstructions (Ferguson, 1984).

Lipase

Lipase is the pancreatic enzyme responsible for changing fats to fatty acids and glycerol. Serum lipase levels are increased after damage of the pancreas occurs.

Lipase levels may not become elevated in acute pancreatitis until 24 to 35 hours after onset. However, lipase levels remain elevated for longer periods (up to 2 weeks) than do amylase levels.

Increased lipase levels also are associated with obstruction of the pancreatic duct, pancreatic carcinoma, acute cholecystitis, cirrhosis, and severe renal disease (Ferguson, 1984).

KIDNEY

The chief function of the kidneys is the production of urine. Another important function of the kidneys is to maintain normal blood pressure. Proper renal function helps to maintain homeostasis — the balance between input/output of water and electrolytes and the acid-base balance of the body.

Some substances cannot be maintained in normal concentrations in the blood in the presence of renal dysfunction. These substances include sodium, potassium, chloride, and urea.

Blood Urea Nitrogen

Urea is the primary nonprotein waste product of protein catabolism. Formed in the liver and transported in the blood to the kidneys, urea normally is excreted in the urine. The blood urea nitrogen (BUN) assay, which measures the nitrogen portion of urea in the blood, is used as a gross index of kidney filtration. Renal dysfunction and rapid protein catabolism will produce elevated BUN levels. The amount of increase depends on the amount of tissue damage sustained, the extent of protein catabolism, and the renal excretion rate of urea nitrogen. Renal dysfunction (caused by kidney disease or failure and urinary obstruction) is the most common cause of an elevated BUN level. Other causes include shock, dehydration, gastrointestinal hemorrhage, diabetes, and infection (Ferguson, 1984).

Creatinine

Creatinine, which is present in skeletal muscle as creatine phosphate, is a by-product of muscle energy production. The amount of creatinine produced is relative to muscle mass. The rate of production remains constant as long as muscle mass remains constant. Removal of creatinine takes place via the blood that transports it to the kidneys. Serum creatinine levels will increase if renal dysfunction (e.g., chronic nephritis, urinary obstruction) impairs creatinine excretion (Ferguson, 1984). Creatinine assays are useful in monitoring renal dysfunction, because they are more sensitive than the BUN assay (Tilkian and Connover, 1975).

Urinalysis

The analysis of urine is performed to detect the presence of the following abnormal substances: red blood cells/casts (hematuria), protein (proteinuria), and elevated levels of white blood cells.

Hematuria is one of the earliest manifestations of renal disease (e.g., acute failure, carcinoma). *Proteinuria* usually results from increased glomerular filtration of protein brought on by renal diseases, including nephritis, polycystic kidney disease, renal stones, renal carcinoma, and ascites. Other causes of proteinuria include fever, trauma, leukemia, and toxemia (Ferguson, 1984). The presence of *large numbers of white blood cells* in the urine usually indicates a urinary tract infection. White blood cell *casts* in urine are associated with acute glomerular nephritis, pyelonephritis, and renal inflammation.

The most common urine test is that for *urinary pH,* which is used as a screening test for renal and respiratory disease and some metabolic disorders. It also is used to monitor diet and drug therapies. In patients with renal calculi, urinary pH is important because the formation of stones partially depends on the pH of urine. The urinary pH can be dietarily adjusted to discourage stone formation. Alkaline urine (pH of 7 or more) is associated with urinary tract infections, chronic renal failure, and pyloric obstruction. Acidic urine (pH of 7 or less) is associated with uncontrolled diabetes, pulmonary emphysema, and dehydration (Tilkian and Connover, 1975).

Another common urine test is that for specific gravity, which tests the kidneys' ability to concentrate urine. The weight of urine is compared to the weight of distilled water (specific gravity 1.00); the normal specific gravity of urine is between 1.003 to 1.035. Diseases that produce low urinary specific gravity include glomerular nephritis, pyelonephritis, renal failure, and diabetes insipidus. Increased specific gravity can result in diabetes mellitus, fever, vomiting, and excessive water loss through diarrhea (Ferguson, 1984). Patient hydration also plays a role in the specific gravity of urine. Large fluid intakes not only increase urinary output but may decrease specific gravity.

HEMATOLOGY

Complete Blood Cell Count

Routine screening of blood includes the following determinations: red blood cell (RBC) count; hematocrit (Hct), hemoglobin (Hgb), white blood cell (WBC) count, and differential white blood cell count (diff). An important additional observation is the sedimentation rate.

Accurate hematologic diagnoses, as well as significant information about disease, can be gathered through the use of blood testing.

Red Blood Cell Count

Red blood cells are formed in the red cell bone marrow. Another term for a mature red blood cell is *erythrocyte.* Erythrocytes, which contain a complex compound called *hemoglobin,* function to transport oxygen to the body cells and to remove carbon dioxide from the cells and transport it to the lungs.

An RBC count refers to the number of red blood cells in one cubic millimeter (cu mm) of blood. Normal values vary for men and women as follows:

For men — 4.2 million to 5.4 million/cu mm
For women — 3.6 million to 5.0 million/cu mm

A decreased RBC count is associated with diseases such as Hodgkin's, leukemia, and hemolytic and pernicious anemias. Increased RBC counts are seen in patients with polycythemia vera and severe diarrhea (Ferguson, 1984).

The total volume of blood that consists of cells is called the *hematocrit*. In this test, which usually is performed on blood removed from the finger, RBCs are separated from the blood plasma. Normal hematocrit values vary, but approximate values are 45 to 47 ml/dl for men and 42 to 44 ml/dl for women. Increased hematocrit values are seen in shock, polycythemia vera, erythrocytosis, and severe dehydration. Decreased values are associated with anemias, leukemia, cirrhosis, and massive blood loss.

White Blood Cell Count

White blood cells (leukocytes) are formed in both the red cell bone marrow and lymphatic tissue. The primary function of WBCs is to control infection through phagocytosis of bacteria and other foreign organisms to produce and distribute antibodies specific to a particular microorganism.

White blood cells are either *granular* or *nongranular*. The granular leukocytes are called *basophils, neutrophils,* and *eosinophils.* The nongranular leukocytes are called *lymphocytes* and *monocytes*. Granulocytes are regulated at a constant level in healthy persons; however, in the presence of infection, their numbers rise dramatically.

The normal WBC count — called the *absolute count* — is about 5000 to 10,000 cells/cu mm. Slight elevations are consistent with 20,000/mm; moderate elevations are considered to be 30,000/cu mm; and marked elevations occur at 50,000/cu mm. A count higher than 10,000/cu mm is called *leukocytosis.* Leukocytosis is associated with acute infections, hemorrhage, carcinoma, and acute leukemias.

The term used to describe a lowered WBC count (below 4000/cu mm) is *leukopenia,* which is associated with hypersplenism, viral infections, leukemia, pernicious and aplastic anemias, and diabetes.

Absolute determination of the leukocytes gives only partial information. Unless an accurate differential WBC count is obtained, a significant pathologic condition or important information can be missed (Tilkian and Connover, 1975).

REFERENCES

Ferguson, G.: Pathophysiology. Mechanisms and Expressions. Philadelphia: W. B. Saunders Co., 1984.

Tilkian, S. M., and Connover, M. H.: Clinical Implications of Laboratory Tests. St. Louis: C. V. Mosby Co., 1975.

▼

A P P E N D I X   5

Acronyms of Professional Organizations

In addition to medical terminology, you should be aware of common organizational acronyms. Those that you will encounter most often in your career in sonography are listed below:

ACC   American College of Cardiology
ACOG   American College of Obstetricians and Gynecologists
ACR   American College of Radiologists
AHA   American Hospital Association
AIUM   American Institute of Ultrasound in Medicine
AMA   American Medical Association
ANA   American Nurses' Association
ARDMS   American Registry of Diagnostic Medical Sonographers
ARRT   American Registry of Radiologic Technologists
ASE   American Society of Echocardiography
ASRT   American Society of Radiologic Technologists
CAHEA   Committee on Allied Health Education and Accreditation
           (AMA)
JCAH   Joint Commission on Accreditation of Hospitals
JRCDMS   Joint Review Committee on Diagnostic Medical Sonography

Index

Note: Page numbers in *italics* indicate illustrations; page numbers followed by t indicate tables.

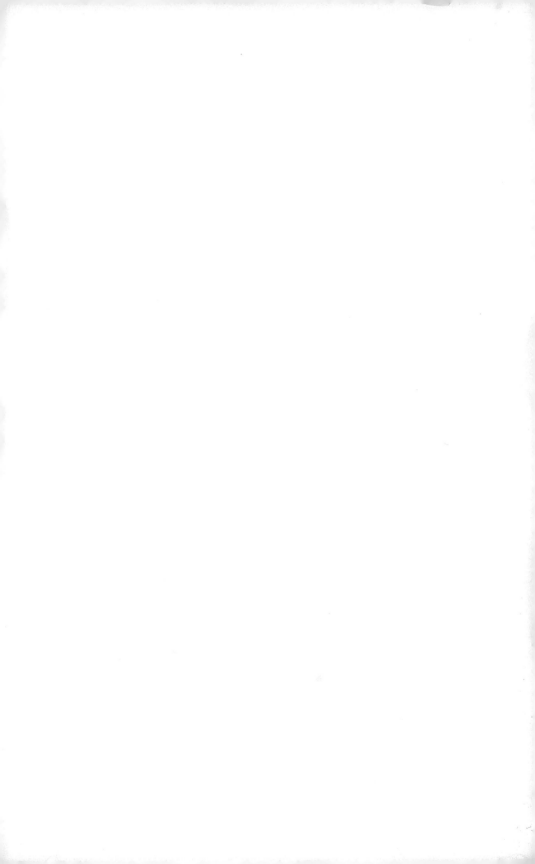